Renal Function : Mechanisms Preserving Fluid and Solute Balance in Health

Plasma osmolality.
= 300 mOsm/kg

Renal Function : Mechanisms Preserving Fluid and Solute Balance in Health

Heinz Valtin, M.D., Andrew C. Vail Professor of Physiology,
Dartmouth Medical School, Hanover, New Hampshire

Little, Brown and Company : Boston

The cover design, representing two kidneys on a background of the world, is based on the official emblem of the V International Congress of Nephrology, Mexico City, 1972. The symbol is used with the kind permission of Dr. Herman Villarreal, President of the Congress.

To
Nancy
and
Tom and Alison

Preface

With the advent of new curricula, virtually every medical educator has had to try to define the basic material in his particular discipline. This book represents my view of the essential elements in renal, fluid, and electrolyte physiology, which every medical student should master. These are necessarily personal choices, and thus most teachers in this field may find some fault with them or, what is more likely, will point out omissions.

Problems. Many chapters are supplemented by one or more quantitative problems that amplify the material in the text. The answers — as well as explanations of how the answers were obtained — are given in the section Answers to Problems following the text.

A note to students. This textbook has been prepared with a certain amount of hesitation, for fear that its concise style may tend to underplay the importance of mastering basic scientific principles. I firmly believe that the basic sciences are the foundation of excellence in medicine. The references at the end of each chapter are meant to underscore this conviction by encouraging those individuals whose curiosity has been aroused to read further. In selecting the references, I have tried to fulfill three purposes: (1) to list some classic contributions; (2) to cite original experiments, especially when their results conflict with those of other studies; and (3) to list review articles in which many further references can be located. As a result, these reference lists, although selective, are somewhat long, and I advise students to enlist the help of their instructors in selecting the particular works that are appropriate to their purpose.

A request for critique. I shall appreciate suggestions from any reader — be he student or teacher — on how this text might be improved.

H. V.

Acknowledgments

Every chapter was reviewed by at least one person who is an expert on the topic treated in that chapter. I shall not name these individuals here, not only because I might inadvertently omit some of them, but also because any errors should not be blamed on them. I trust that I have thanked them all personally for their very real help.

I am grateful to many authors and publishers for permission to reproduce their work. I have tried to acknowledge this debt — especially in the case of original photographs — in the legends to the figures.

Special thanks are due Mrs. Grace E. McCann for her invariably cheerful patience in typing the manuscript, from first draft to final copy. Mrs. Ethel B. Garrity kindly proofread the entire manuscript. Valma and Henry Page and Genevieve Zyskowski diligently prepared all the illustrations. The librarians of the Dana Biomedical Library at Dartmouth College provided an amiable atmosphere and much thoughtful and expert help. It was a real pleasure to work with the superb staff at Little, Brown and Company through all phases of production.

Finally, I was greatly aided by the on-the-spot advice of a number of colleagues at Dartmouth Medical School, especially S. Marsh Tenney, Gilbert H. Mudge, William O. Berndt, John T. Gatzy, Howard H. Green, and Richard D. Mamelok.

H. V.

Contents

Renal Function : Mechanisms Preserving Fluid and Solute Balance in Health

1 : Components of Renal Function

The lay view of renal function is that the kidneys remove waste liquids and potentially harmful end products of metabolism, such as urea, uric acid, sulfates, and phosphates. While this is true, it should be emphasized that an equally important function is the conservation of substances that are essential to life. Such substances include water, sugars, amino acids, and electrolytes such as sodium, potassium, bicarbonate, and chloride. Therefore, the kidneys should be viewed as regulatory organs that selectively excrete and conserve water and numerous chemical compounds and thereby help to preserve the constancy of the internal environment.

A castaway at sea may survive for three weeks without drinking water, and a man lost in the desert may survive from two to four days without water or salt. Conversely, a healthy individual frequently tolerates dietary excesses of fluid and salt. The reason that such extreme conditions can be endured lies primarily in the renal control of salt and water excretion and conservation. It is obvious that the renal adjustments must be relatively rapid if they are to preserve life. In fact they are brought into play within minutes or at most a few hours after the individual has been subjected to the environmental challenge.

Anatomy

The major gross anatomical features of the mammalian kidney are illustrated in Figure 1-1. The kidney consists of cortical and medullary substances and a pelvis that connects with the ureter. The medullary substance is divided into an outer and inner zone (Fig. 1-2a), the latter comprising one or more papillae, depending on the species. The renal artery enters the kidney alongside the ureter, branching to become progressively the interlobar artery, the arciform or arcuate artery, the interlobular artery, and then the afferent arteriole that leads to the glomerular capillary network. The venous system has subdivisions with similar designations, terminating in the renal vein, which also courses beside the ureter.

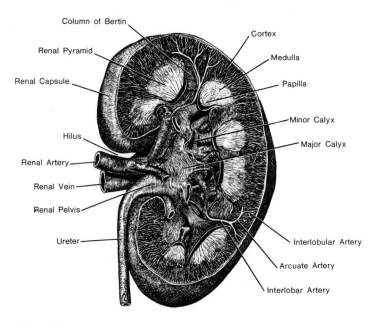

Column of Bertin

Renal Pyramid

Renal Capsule

Hilus

Renal Artery

Renal Vein

Renal Pelvis

Ureter

Cortex

Medulla

Papilla

Minor Calyx

Major Calyx

Interlobular Artery

Arcuate Artery

Interlobar Artery

Figure 1-1
Sagittal section of a human kidney, showing the major gross anatomical features. The renal columns are extensions of cortical tissue between the medullary areas. Redrawn and very slightly modified from Braus, H. *Anatomie des Menschen*, vol. 2. Springer, Berlin, 1924.

By *renal blood flow* (RBF), we mean the total amount of blood that traverses either the renal artery or the renal vein per unit time. The difference between flow in the renal artery and flow in the vein is the urine flow, which is negligibly small compared to the total blood flow. In adult man about 1,300 ml of blood (i.e., about 25% of the cardiac output) flows through the two kidneys each minute, even though they constitute less than 0.5% of the total body weight. About 1,299 ml of blood leaves through the renal veins each minute, so a normal urine flow is about 1 ml per minute. *Renal plasma flow* (RPF) refers to the amount of plasma that traverses either the renal artery or the renal vein per unit time. Obviously, if the systemic hematocrit is 45%, RPF constitutes 55% of RBF.

The Nephron

The nephron, or functional unit of the kidney, consists of a glomerular capillary network that is surrounded by Bowman's capsule, a proximal convoluted tubule, a loop of Henle, a distal convoluted tubule, and a collecting duct (Fig. 1-2a). Together, the adult human kidneys comprise roughly two million such functional units, which provide tremendous reserve. Man at rest can survive on about one-tenth this amount of functioning renal tissue, and he can continue an active life even though about 75% of the tissue has been destroyed.

Superficial Cortical and Juxtamedullary Nephrons. As is illustrated in Figure 1-2(a) and (b), two types of nephron have been described. The superficial cortical nephron has a short loop of Henle that reaches varying distances into the outer medulla, and its efferent arteriole branches into the peritubular capillary network that surrounds the tubular segments belonging to its own and other nephrons. This capillary network nourishes the tubular cells, picks up substances that have been reabsorbed from the tubules, and brings substances to the tubules for secretion.

The juxtamedullary nephron arises from the deep cortical regions. Its glomerulus is larger than that of a superficial cortical nephron, and its loop of Henle extends varying distances into the inner medulla, sometimes all the way to the papillary tip. Its efferent arteriole continues not only as a peritubular capillary network but also as a series of vascular loops called the vasa recta. The vasa recta descend in bundles to varying depths in the inner medulla, or papilla. There they break up into capillary networks that surround the collecting ducts and ascending limbs of Henle. The blood then returns to the cortex in ascending vasa recta that run within the vascular bundles. The ratio of superficial cortical to juxtamedullary nephrons varies with the species of mammal. In man, about seven-eighths of all nephrons are superficial cortical and one-eighth are juxtamedullary.

Ultrastructural Differences of Various Nephron Segments. Epithelial cells lining the various nephron segments differ in many respects, such as size, number and length of microvilli at the apical (mucosal) surface, number of mitochondria, number and extent of basal infoldings, and many others. The major differences are shown in Figure 1-3. Although the functional significance of some of these variations has not yet been clarified, many fruitful correlations between structure and function have been drawn, and these will be referred to when appropriate.

The Juxtaglomerular Apparatus (JGA)

This apparatus (Fig. 1-3) consists of specialized epithelial cells in the very early distal tubule, the macula densa cells, and specialized secretory or granular cells at the vascular pole where the afferent and efferent arterioles enter and leave the glomerulus. The JGA thus is a combination of specialized tubular and vascular cells. The macula densa cells always come into intimate

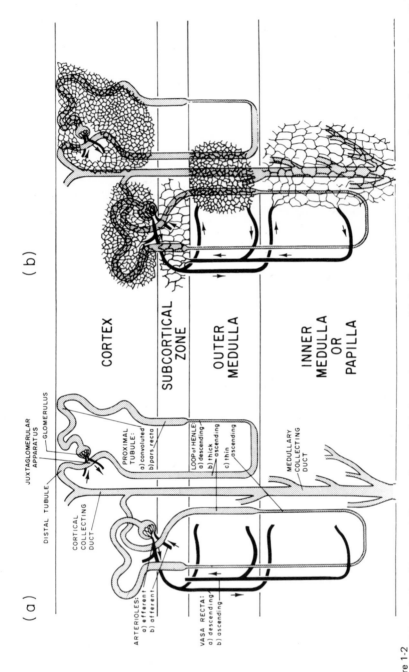

Figure 1-2

(a) Superficial cortical and juxtamedullary nephrons, and their vasculature. The glomerulus plus the surrounding Bowman's capsule are known as the "renal corpuscle." The beginning of the proximal tubule — the so-called urinary pole — lies opposite the vascular pole, where the afferent and efferent arterioles enter and leave the glomerulus. The early distal tubule is always closely associated with the vascular pole belonging to the same nephron; the juxtaglomerular apparatus is located at the point of contact.

(b) Capillary networks have been superimposed on the nephrons illustrated in (a). Note that the capillary network that is interposed between descending and ascending vasa recta surrounds primarily the collecting duct and the ascending limb of Henle. In the outer and inner medulla, the vasa recta run in bundles, closely associated with the descending limb of Henle. Parts (a) and (b), slightly modified, are from Kriz, W., and Lever, A. F. *Amer. Heart J.* 78:101, 1969.

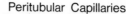

Peritubular Capillaries

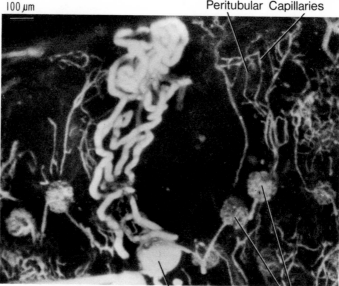

Renal Corpuscle   Glomeruli

(c) The cortex of a dog kidney (photomicrograph) illustrating the highly convoluted course of the proximal tubule. A micropipet (white streak at the lower left) was inserted into Bowman's space, and the convolutions were filled with a silicone rubber compound ("Microfil"). Other glomeruli, as well as peritubular capillaries, were partially filled with Microfil through an intra-arterial injection. Photograph courtesy of R. Beeuwkes and A. C. Barger.

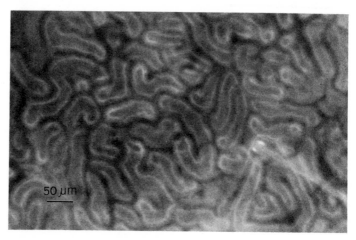

50 μm

(d) The surface of a rat kidney as seen during micropuncture. The so-called bag of worms consists mainly of segments of proximal convolutions as they repeatedly rise to the surface. A few segments of distal convolutions are also visible, but glomeruli are not usually found at the surface of a mammalian kidney. Each tubular segment is surrounded by peritubular capillaries. The light, linear streak in the lower right is a micropipet that has been inserted into a tubular segment. The pipet is out of focus because its shaft lies above the renal surface. Photograph courtesy of J. Schnermann.

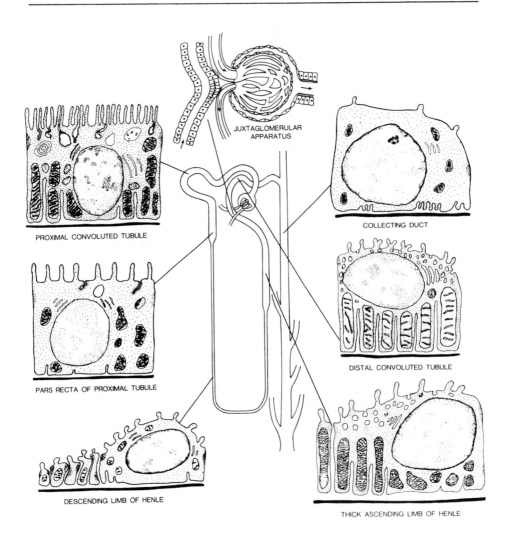

Figure 1-3
Diagrams illustrating some of the ultrastructural differences of the major segments of the nephron. Also shown is the juxtaglomerular apparatus, which lies at the point of contact between the distal tubule and the vascular pole of its own glomerulus. Adapted from Rhodin, J. *Int. Rev. Cytology* 7:485, 1958.

contact with the granular cells of the arterioles belonging to the same nephron; this is the result of embryonic development, not of some magic process whereby the distal tubule seeks out its own glomerulus. The JGA is thought to secrete renin, which is involved in the formation of angiotensin and ultimately in the secretion of aldosterone. It has been postulated that the JGA may be part of a feedback system that accounts for the autoregulation of the glomerular filtration rate and the renal blood flow, a topic that is considered further in Chapter 6.

Processes Involved in the Formation of Urine

The anatomical arrangement of the nephron permits several theories of function; these were hotly debated until the true picture emerged about 50 years ago. In 1842, William Bowman proposed that the glomerular capillaries secrete water, which flushes out solutes secreted by the renal tubules, a view elaborated about 40 years later by Heidenhain. In 1844, Carl Ludwig stated that urine is formed by ultrafiltration of plasma at the glomerulus, and that it merely passes down the nephron without further alteration save for concentration of its solutes by passive reabsorption of water. In 1917, Arthur Cushny modified Ludwig's view by proposing that not only water but also solutes are reabsorbed by the tubules, in "proportions, which are determined by their normal values in the plasma." Cushny denied the possibility of selective tubular secretion because he thought it was a process that would require vitalistic discrimination. It was not until 1923 that E. K. Marshall, Jr., proved that tubular secretion occurs.

We now know that the formation of urine involves a combination of ultrafiltration at the glomerulus, followed by selective tubular reabsorption of water and solutes, and selective tubular secretion of solutes. The subject of renal physiology deals primarily with defining what substances are filtered, reabsorbed, and secreted, in what amounts, in which parts of the nephron, by what mechanisms, and to what purpose.

Magnitude of Renal Function

The tremendous amounts of water and of certain solutes that are handled by the kidneys every day are illustrated in Table 1-1. The quantities that are filtered become even more astonishing when one considers that the total amount of water in adult man is about 42 liters, and his pool of readily exchangeable sodium about 3,000 mEq. This disparity between total availability of essential substances and the rates at which they are filtered points

Table 1-1
Daily renal turnover of H_2O, Na^+, HCO_3^-, and Cl^- in adult man.

		Filtered	Excreted	Reabsorbed	Proportion of Filtered Load That Is Reabsorbed (%)
H_2O	L/day	180	1.5	178.5	99.2
Na^+	mEq/day	25,000	150	24,850	99.4
HCO_3^-	mEq/day	4,500	2	4,498	99.9+
Cl^-	mEq/day	18,000	150	17,850	99.2

up the necessity for their conservation through reabsorption. Since the examples listed in Table 1-1, as well as many others, are critical components of the internal environment, it is not surprising that they are reabsorbed so avidly. What may be surprising is that the kidneys should operate in such a seemingly inefficient manner as to filter the substances in the first place. The answer to this apparent paradox probably lies in the evolution of renal function.

Evolution

One possible scheme for the evolution of the kidney is depicted in Figure 1-4. The prochordate ancestor of the vertebrates, such as the acorn worm, may have evolved in the Cambrian Sea about 550 million years ago. These animals drank the sea water, bathed their tissues in it, and then expelled the residue through a simple ciliated conduit, which may be the forerunner of the kidney. The Cambrian Sea may have had a relatively high NaCl concentration similar to that of present-day mammalian extracellular fluid (Chap. 2). As fish migrated into fresh water, they retained an internal environment of high salinity, so that their body fluids had a higher osmolality than the freshwater surroundings. The consequent osmotic flow of water into these fish could have resulted in fatal swelling unless an organ capable of high rates of water excretion had been evolved through natural selection. This organ was the glomerulus, promoting the ultrafiltration of large amounts of plasma, about 92% of which is water. The filtered plasma, however, also contained essential small molecules (often referred to as crystalloids), such as sodium, chloride, bicarbonate, sugars, and amino acids. These essentials were reabsorbed in the proximal tubules, along with osmotically obligated water. The

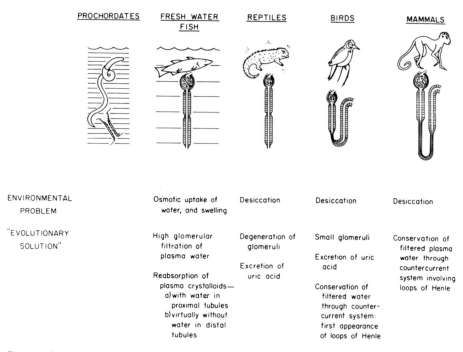

PROCHORDATES	FRESH WATER FISH	REPTILES	BIRDS	MAMMALS
ENVIRONMENTAL PROBLEM	Osmotic uptake of water, and swelling	Desiccation	Desiccation	Desiccation
"EVOLUTIONARY SOLUTION"	High glomerular filtration of plasma water Reabsorption of plasma crystalloids— a) with water in proximal tubules b) virtually without water in distal tubules	Degeneration of glomeruli Excretion of uric acid	Small glomeruli Excretion of uric acid Conservation of filtered water through counter-current system: first appearance of loops of Henle	Conservation of filtered plasma water through countercurrent system involving loops of Henle

Figure 1-4

One possible scheme for the evolution of the vertebrate kidney. Modified from: Pitts, R. F. *Physiology of the Kidney and Body Fluids,* 2d ed. Year Book, Chicago, 1968; and Smith, H. W. *The Evolution of the Kidney.* Porter Lectures, Series IX, University of Kansas Press, Lawrence, 1943. Pp. 1—23. It should be noted that J. D. Robertson, among others, does not agree with this scheme. He has proposed that glomerular kidneys may have existed in marine protovertebrates, and that they thus may have been a useful preadaptation for life in fresh water.

need to expel water may have been so great that a new structure evolved, namely the distal tubule, in which the small molecules could be reabsorbed to the virtual exclusion of water.

When the vertebrates migrated onto land, they faced the opposite problem of the freshwater fish: desiccation. The consequent need to conserve water was apparently solved in two ways: In reptiles, the process of filtration was reduced through evolutionary degeneration of the glomerulus, and uric acid became the excretory end product of protein catabolism. In contrast to urea, which is the main nitrogenous end product of mammals, uric acid can exist in highly supersaturated solutions and can thus be excreted with minimal amounts of water. In mammals, on the other hand, glomeruli of high filtering capacity were retained, as was the ability to recover essential small molecules mainly in the proximal tubules. In addition, selective forces apparently led to the development of loops of Henle, which promote the avid conservation of water through the countercurrent system (Chap. 8). It is of considerable interest that birds exhibit both solutions, excreting uric acid and also having some loops of Henle.

Summary

The kidneys are regulatory organs that help to maintain constancy of the internal environment in regard to both its volume and composition. They accomplish this purpose through ultrafiltration of plasma at the glomerulus, selective reabsorption of water and solutes, and selective tubular secretion of solutes. The objective of renal physiology is to understand the mechanisms, both within and outside of the kidneys, by which the renal regulation of fluid and solute balance is accomplished. Many special features of renal function, such as the very high rate of blood flow in relation to its size, the difference in both structure and function of the nephron depending on its location within the kidney, and the apparent inefficiency of concurrent, high rates of filtration and reabsorption, may be understood through the evolutionary forces that selected for ability to preserve water and solute balance.

Selected References

General

Berliner, R. W. (Ed.). Symposium on the kidney. *Amer. J. Med.* 36:641, 1964.

Chasis, H., and Goldring, W. (Eds.). *Homer William Smith: His Scientific and Literary Achievements.* New York University Press, New York, 1965.

Cohen, J. J. Renal Metabolism of Substrates in Relation to Renal Function. In J. Orloff and R. W. Berliner (Eds.), *Handbook of Physiology.* Section 8: Renal Physiology. American Physiological Society, Washington, D.C., 1973.

Fisher, J. W. (Ed.). *Kidney Hormones.* Academic, New York, 1971.

Forster, R. P. Comparative Vertebrate Physiology and Renal Concepts. In J. Orloff and R. W. Berliner (Eds.), *Handbook of Physiology.* Section 8: Renal Physiology. American Physiological Society, Washington, D.C., 1973.

Kiil, F., and Setekliev, J. Physiology of Ureter and Renal Pelvis. In J. Orloff and R. W. Berliner (Eds.), *Handbook of Physiology.* Section 8: Renal Physiology. American Physiological Society, Washington, D.C., 1973.

Lotspeich, W. D. *Metabolic Aspects of Renal Function.* Thomas, Springfield, Ill., 1959.

Mudge, G. H., and Taggart, J. V. (Eds.). Symposium on renal physiology. *Amer. J. Med.* 24:659, 1958.

Orloff, J., and Berliner, R. W. (Eds.). *Handbook of Physiology.* Section 8: Renal Physiology. American Physiological Society, Washington, D.C., 1973.

Pitts, R. F. *Physiology of the Kidney and Body Fluids,* 2d ed. Year Book, Chicago, 1968.

Seldin, D. W. (Guest Ed.). Special issue dedicated to Dr. Robert F. Pitts. *Nephron* 6:161, 1969.

Smith, H. W. *Lectures on the Kidney.* Porter Lectures, Series IX. University Extension Division, University of Kansas, Lawrence, 1943.

Smith, H. W. *The Kidney: Structure and Function in Health and Disease.* Oxford University Press, New York, 1951.

Wesson, L. G. *Physiology of the Human Kidney.* Grune & Stratton, New York, 1969.

Winton, F. R. (Ed.). *Modern Views on the Secretion of Urine.* Churchill, London, 1956.

Anatomy and
Development

Barajas, L., and Latta, H. Structure of the juxtaglomerular apparatus. *Circ. Res.* 21(Suppl. II):II-15, 1967.

Bulger, R. E., Tisher, C. C., Meyers, C. H., and Trump, B. F. Human renal ultrastructure: II. The thin limb of Henle's loop and the interstitium in healthy individuals. *Lab. Invest.* 16:124, 1967.

Dalton, A. J., and Haguenau, F. (Eds.). *Ultrastructure of the Kidney.* Academic, New York, 1967.

Fourman, J., and Moffat, D. B. *The Blood Vessels of the Kidney.* Blackwell, Oxford, 1972.

Huber, G. C. On the development and shape of uriniferous tubules of certain of the higher mammals. *Amer. J. Anat.* 4(Suppl. 1):1, 1905.

Kriz, W. Der architektonische und funktionelle Aufbau der Rattenniere. *Ztschr. Zellforschung* 82:495, 1967.

Latta, H., and Maunsbach, A. B. The juxtaglomerular apparatus as studied electron microscopically. *J. Ultrastruct. Res.* 6:547, 1962.

Maunsbach, A. B. Ultrastructure of the Proximal Tubule. In J. Orloff and R. W. Berliner (Eds.), *Handbook of Physiology.* Section 8: Renal Physiology. American Physiological Society, Washington, D.C., 1973.

von Möllendorff, W.   Der Exkretionsapparat. In W. von Möllendorff (Ed.), *Handbuch der Mikroskopischen Anatomie des Menschen,* vol. VII, part 1. Springer, Berlin, 1930.

Oliver, J.   *Nephrons and Kidneys: A Quantitative Study of Developmental and Evolutionary Mammalian Architectonics.* Harper & Row, New York, 1968.

Osathanondth, V., and Potter, E. L.   Development of human kidney as shown by microdissection. (This is a series of five papers by these authors, all published in *Arch. Path.*, as follows: I. 76:271, 1963; II. 76:277, 1963; III. 76:290, 1963; IV. 82:391, 1966; V. 82:403, 1966.)

Peter, K.   *Untersuchungen über Bau und Entwickelung der Niere.* Fischer, Jena, 1909.

Rollhäuser, H., Kriz, W., and Heinke, W.   Das Gefäss-system der Rattenniere. *Ztschr. Zellforschung* 64:381, 1964.

Rouiller, C., and Muller, A. F. (Eds.).   *The Kidney,* vol. I. Academic, New York, 1969.

Rytand, D. A.   The number and size of mammalian glomeruli as related to kidney and to body weight, with methods for their enumeration and measurement. *Amer. J. Anat.* 62:507, 1938.

Sperber, I.   Studies on the mammalian kidney. *Zool. Bid. Fran. Uppsala.* 22:249, 1944.

Thoenes, W., and Langer, K. H.   Relationship Between Cell Structures of Renal Tubules and Transport Mechanisms. In K. Thurau and H. Jahrmärker (Eds.), *Renal Transport and Diuretics.* Springer, New York, 1969.

Tisher, C. C., Bulger, R. E., and Trump, B. F.   Human renal ultrastructure: I. Proximal tubule of healthy individuals. *Lab. Invest.* 15:1357, 1966.

Tisher, C. C., Bulger, R. E., and Trump, B. F.   Human renal ultrastructure: III. The distal tubule in healthy individuals. *Lab. Invest.* 18:655, 1968.

Trump, B. F., and Bulger, R. E.   Morphology of the Kidney. In E. L. Becker (Ed.), *Structural Basis of Renal Disease.* Harper & Row, New York, 1968.

Historical

Bowman, W.   On the structure and use of the malpighian bodies of the kidney, with observations on the circulation through that gland. *Phil. Trans. Roy. Soc. London* 132:57, 1842.

Cushny, A. R.   *The Secretion of Urine.* Longmans, Green, London, 1917.

Heidenhain, R. Die Harnabsonderung. In L. Hermann (Ed.), *Handbuch der Physiologie,* vol. V, part 1. Vogel, Leipzig, 1883.

Ludwig, C. Nieren und Harnbereitung. In R. Wagner (Ed.), *Handwörterbuch der Physiologie.* Vieweg, Braunschweig, 1844.

Marshall, E. K., Jr., and Vickers, J. L. The mechanism of the elimination of phenolsulphonphthalein by the kidney — proof of secretion by the convoluted tubules. *Johns Hopkins Bull.* 34:1, 1923.

Evolution

Robertson, J. D. The habitat of the early vertebrates. *Biol. Rev.* 32:156, 1957.

Smith, H. W. *The Evolution of the Kidney.* Porter Lectures, Series IX. University of Kansas Press, Lawrence, 1943.

Smith, H. W. *From Fish to Philosopher.* Little, Brown, Boston, 1953.

Research Techniques

Burg, M., and Orloff, J. Perfusion of Isolated Renal Tubules. In J. Orloff and R. W. Berliner (Eds.), *Handbook of Physiology.* Section 8: Renal Physiology. American Physiological Society, Washington, D.C., 1973.

Gottschalk, C. W. *Renal Tubular Function: Lessons from Micropuncture.* Harvey Lectures, Series LVIII, 1962–63. Academic, New York, 1963.

Gottschalk, C. W., and Lassiter, W. E. Micropuncture Methodology. In J. Orloff and R. W. Berliner (Eds.), *Handbook of Physiology.* Section 8: Renal Physiology. American Physiological Society, Washington, D.C., 1973.

Levinsky, N. G., and Levy, M. Clearance Techniques. In J. Orloff and R. W. Berliner (Eds.), *Handbook of Physiology.* Section 8: Renal Physiology. American Physiological Society, Washington, D.C., 1973.

Malvin, R. L., and Wilde, W. S. Stop-flow Technique. In J. Orloff and R. W. Berliner (Eds.), *Handbook of Physiology.* Section 8: Renal Physiology. American Physiological Society, Washington, D.C., 1973.

Richards, A. N. *Urine Formation in the Amphibian Kidney.* Harvey Lectures, Series XXX, 1934–35. Williams & Wilkins, Baltimore, 1936.

Walker, A., Bott, P., Oliver, J., and MacDowell, M. The collection and analysis of fluid from single nephrons of the mammalian kidney. *Amer. J. Physiol.* 134:580, 1941.

Wearn, J. T., and Richards, A. N. Observations on the composition of glomerular urine with particular reference to the problem of reabsorption in the renal tubules. *Amer. J. Physiol.* 71:209, 1924.

Windhager, E. E. *Micropuncture Techniques and Nephron Function.* Appleton-Century-Crofts, New York, 1968.

2 : The Body Fluid Compartments

The internal environment that is regulated by the kidneys is a fluid medium, which is distributed in a number of discernible compartments. In this chapter, we shall consider both the size and the distinctive composition of these compartments, as well as some of the factors that maintain these characteristic differences.

Size of the Compartments

Approximate sizes of the major fluid compartments of adult man are shown in Figure 2-1, where the dimensions have been expressed both as absolute values and as a proportion of the body weight. The latter is important because it is one basis for estimating fluid volumes, both in experimental animals and in patients. It should be emphasized that all percentages refer to the proportion of *body weight,* not of total body water.

About 50 to 70% of the body is composed of water. The main factor that determines whether the lower or higher figure applies is the amount of fatty tissue, which has a low water content compared to other tissues. Thus, the lower figure pertains mainly to obese individuals, and to females who have relatively more fat than men.

The total body water (TBW) is distributed between two major compartments, the intracellular (ICW) and the extracellular (ECW). Of these, ICW is the larger, comprising nearly two-thirds of the TBW. The ECW has two further major subdivisions, the plasma and the interstitial, comprising about 4% and 16% of the body weight, respectively. Lymph, constituting 2 to 3% of the body weight, is included in the interstitial volume. Claude Bernard first pointed out that of all the body fluid compartments, the interstitial is probably the true internal environment, since it is the fluid medium that bathes all cells.

The transcellular compartment is a minor subdivision of ECW. It comprises a number of small volumes, such as cerebrospinal, intraocular, pleural, peritoneal, and synovial fluids, and the digestive secretions. Unlike interstitial fluid, the transcellular

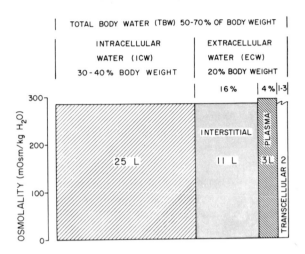

Figure 2-1
Approximate sizes of the major body fluid compartments, expressed both as percentage of body weight and in mean absolute values for an adult human being who weighs 70 kg (154 lb). The ranges of normal among individuals are considerable, and thus no one value should be taken too rigidly. The plasma has a slightly higher osmolality than the intracellular and interstitial compartments; this small difference can be ignored when dealing with problems of fluid balance.

spaces are separated from the blood not only by capillary endothelium but also by epithelium. Except in special circumstances, such as loss of gastrointestinal fluid, the transcellular compartment may be neglected in experimental and clinical problems of fluid balance.

Relationship of Tissue Water to Tissue Volume

The terms *intracellular, interstitial,* and *plasma "water"* are commonly used interchangeably with the corresponding "fluid" or "volume." Although this is not accurate, in most instances it is permissible for practical purposes, since the vast proportion of each compartment is water. Water constitutes about 94% of the plasma compartment, while for most intracellular spaces the value is 75 to 80%. Bone cells and fat cells, with about 20% and 10% of water, respectively, are notable exceptions.

Measuring the Size of Compartments

Total Body Water. These measurements all involve the simple principle of dilution, usually of a substance that can be measured colorimetrically, or of a radioactively labeled compound. For example, TBW can be estimated with a drug, antipyrine, which distributes itself quickly throughout all the major fluid compartments, or with heavy water, D_2O, or tritiated water, HTO. The following is an illustration using tritiated water.

An adult woman who weighs 60 kg is given exactly 1 millicurie (mCi) of HTO intravenously. On the basis of prior experiments in humans, it is known that within 2 hours after the injection, this labeled water will have come into equilibrium with interstitial and intracellular water, and that by this time about 0.4% of the administered dose will have been lost from the internal environment, mainly via the urine. At this time, therefore, a plasma sample is withdrawn and its radioactivity measured by liquid scintillation; it is found to be 0.031 mCi per liter of plasma water. From the relationship:

$$\text{Concentration} = \frac{\text{Amount}}{\text{Volume}} \qquad (2\text{-}1)$$

and knowing that the concentration of HTO in the major compartments will be the same as in plasma, the TBW will therefore be:

$$\frac{0.031 \text{ mCi}}{1{,}000 \text{ ml plasma water}} = \frac{1 \text{ mCi} - (1 \cdot 0.004)}{\text{TBW}}$$

TBW = 32,129 ml, or about 32 liters. Thus, the general equation for measuring a volume by the dilution principle is:

$$\frac{\text{Volume of}}{\text{compartment}} = \frac{\text{Amount of substance X given} - \text{Amount of X lost from compartment}}{\text{Concentration of X in the compartment}} \qquad (2\text{-}2)$$

The final volume has been deliberately stated as "about" 32 liters because the method may yield an estimate that is high by perhaps 1 liter. The discrepancy arises mainly from exchange of the isotope with hydrogen atoms of organic molecules.

Extracellular Water. The substances and equations used to measure the size of the various compartments are summarized in Table 2-1. There is no ideal test substance for estimating ECW because all substances that diffuse freely from the vascular into the interstitial compartment also in small part penetrate cells; for example, chloride ions enter erythrocytes and are secreted as gastric juice, two losses that are difficult to quantify.

Plasma. This compartment is measured by the dilution of substances that distribute themselves almost exclusively within

Table 2-1
Substances and equations used to measure the size of the major body fluid compartments.

Compartment	Substance	Equation
TBW	Antipyrine	2-2
	D_2O	
	HTO	
ECW	Inulin	2-2
	Raffinose	
	Sucrose	
	Mannitol	
	Thiosulfate	
	Radiosulfate	
	Thiocyanate	
	Radiochloride	
	Radiosodium	
Plasma	^{131}I-albumin	2-2
	Evans blue, or T-1824	
	^{51}Cr-erythrocytes	
Interstitial	Not measured directly	Interstitial = ECW — Plasma
ICW	Not measured directly	ICW = TBW — ECW

the plasma. Radioiodinated serum albumin falls short of the ideal substance in that some albumin crosses the capillary endothelium into the interstitial space. The same shortcoming applies to the dye known as Evans blue (T-1824), which is bound to serum albumin and thus has the same volume of distribution as the protein. Tagged erythrocytes yield a slightly inaccurate result because erythrocytes do not distribute themselves evenly throughout the plasma; the hematocrit (i.e., the ratio of the volume of blood cells to that of plasma) is less in fine, peripheral vessels than it is in large, major vessels.

Interstitial and Intracellular Water.   These volumes are not measured directly because there are no known substances that distribute themselves exclusively within these compartments. They are thus calculated as the difference between two compartments that were measured by the dilution technique. The formulas are given in Table 2-1; their derivation is self-evident, or can be deduced from Figure 2-1.

Body Weight. In many circumstances, changes in body weight provide the most accurate estimate of a change in TBW. As has been mentioned, the measurement of TBW by the dilution technique involves an error of about 1,000 ml in an adult human. The body weight can be determined much more accurately, simply, and cheaply. And in an experimental animal or patient who is eating adequately, an acute change in body weight will be due almost solely to a change in TBW. Of course, this measurement cannot tell us which of the body fluid compartments has lost or gained water, but this additional information can often be surmised from the history of an illness or experimental situation.

The usefulness of measuring body weight in the field of fluid and solute balance cannot be overemphasized, and it will be referred to repeatedly in this book. Too many physicians tend to forget that this simple measure frequently yields more accurate and immediate information than do the cumbersome and expensive dilution methods.

Composition of the Compartments

The main solute constituents of the major body fluid compartments are shown in Figure 2-2. Note that these compartments are made up primarily of electrolytes. Although the conveyance by these fluids of nutrients and waste products such as glucose, amino acids, and urea is very important, the nonelectrolytes constitute only a small portion of the total solute.

The concentrations have been expressed as chemical equivalents. Although there is an electrical potential difference (P.D.) at the interface between the compartments, the separation of charges is confined to the immediate area of the interface and involves only a minute fraction of the total number of ions. Hence, the bulk of the fluid within a compartment is electrically neutral. The total number of equivalents varies, however, from one compartment to another. As Figure 2-2 clearly shows, this difference is due to the variation in the concentration of proteins. At the pH of body fluids, proteins have multiple negative charges per molecule. Hence intracellular fluid, being relatively rich in proteins, has more total charges than does extracellular fluid. The same explanation applies to the greater total equivalents in plasma as opposed to interstitial fluid.

Sodium is by far the most abundant cation of vertebrate extracellular fluid, and chloride and bicarbonate are the most abundant anions. In contrast, potassium is the most plentiful intracellular cation, and organic phosphates and proteins are the

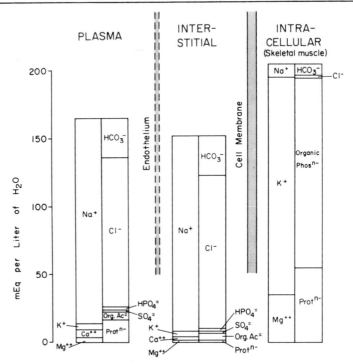

Figure 2-2
The main solute constituents of the major body fluid compartments. The concentrations are expressed as chemical equivalents to emphasize that the compartments are made up mainly of electrolytes, and that within any one space the total number of negative charges is neutralized by the positive charges.

The values depicted for intracellular fluid are rough approximations at best. They reflect current estimates for skeletal muscle, but since some cells have unique composition, these estimates are not precisely representative of all intracellular fluid. Furthermore, the extent to which some intracellular ions are bound or ionized is not known, so that the equivalences for such ions, as well as for organic phosphates and proteins, are also approximations. Despite these limitations, however, the diagram serves to emphasize important and typical differences between intracellular and extracellular fluid. Organic phosphates include AMP, ADP, and ATP, glycerophosphate, and creatine phosphate. Slightly modified from Gamble, J. L. *Chemical Anatomy, Physiology and Pathology of Extracellular Fluid,* 6th ed. Harvard University Press, Cambridge, 1954.

major anions. The similarity in composition between plasma and interstitial fluid is striking, and is explained by the fact that these two compartments are separated by a semipermeable membrane, the capillary endothelium, which allows free diffusion of solutes of low molecular weight (often referred to as "crystalloids").

Explanation for
Differences
in Composition

The main difference between plasma and interstitial fluid is in the concentration of proteins, which are largely excluded from the interstitial compartment by the capillary endothelium. In conformity with the Gibbs-Donnan relationship (see below), there is a difference of about 5% in the concentrations of diffusible ions between the two compartments. The concentrations of cations are slightly greater in plasma than they are in the interstitial fluid; the concentrations of diffusible anions are slightly smaller in plasma than they are in the interstitial fluid. Thus, the differences in composition between plasma and interstitial fluid can be accounted for almost entirely by the unequal distribution of proteins and the resultant Gibbs-Donnan equilibrium. Binding of certain cations, such as calcium and magnesium, to proteins makes a further, small contribution to the differences.

The intracellular compartment is separated from interstitial fluid by the cell membrane (Fig. 2-2). This barrier, unlike the endothelium, has selective permeabilities not only for proteins but also for certain other ions such as the organic phosphates. In addition, the membrane of most cells has a "pump" or pumps that extrude sodium from the cells and move potassium into them. Net movement of these ions across the membrane is called "active" because it requires energy; for example, when a cellular system is exposed to a metabolic poison such as dinitrophenol (DNP), the cells gain sodium and lose potassium (Fig. 2-6). Of course, since most of the intracellular anions are barred from interstitial fluid by the cell membrane, the Gibbs-Donnan effect also applies, and may largely account for the low intracellular concentrations of bicarbonate and chloride. Finally, there is probably considerable binding of certain ions to intracellular proteins and phosphates. Thus, the striking compositional differences between extracellular and intracellular fluids result from the combined effects of selective permeabilities, metabolic pumps, Gibbs-Donnan forces, and ion-binding.

Osmolality in the Major Compartments

It has been shown by a number of experimental techniques that the osmolality of interstitial fluid is equal to that of intracellular fluid (Fig. 2-1). It should be noted that this fact is not in conflict with the differences in total equivalents depicted in Figure 2-2. Osmolality is a function of the *number* of discrete particles in solution (Chap. 7). Thus, a single atom of sodium contributes as much to the osmolality of a solution as does a single molecule of protein, even though the latter weighs perhaps 3,000 times more than the former. But at the pH of body fluids, each molecule of protein contributes several charges to the total equivalence, whereas each atom of sodium contributes only one charge. If the interstitial and intracellular concentrations in Figure 2-2 were expressed as millimoles per liter of H_2O and the proper dissociation constants were applied to each compound, such as NaCl or $NaHCO_3$ the resulting osmolalities in the interstitial and intracellular compartments would be equal, as is shown in Figure 2-1.

Note that the osmolality of plasma is slightly higher than that of interstitial and intracellular fluid. This difference has not been demonstrated directly, since neither interstitial nor intracellular fluid can be sampled; however, according to the Gibbs-Donnan equilibrium (see below), the difference must exist. Its magnitude is not known; it may amount to perhaps 10 mOsm per kilogram H_2O, and it is usually ignored when dealing with experimental or clinical problems of fluid balance. This fact has often led to the erroneous statement that *all* the major fluid compartments are osmotically equilibrated; this is not true of plasma, although in solving problems of fluid balance one treats the plasma *as if* it were in osmotic equilibrium with interstitial and intracellular fluid. This simplification does not introduce serious errors.

Gibbs-Donnan Equilibrium

This equilibrium explains the unequal distribution of diffusible ions on the two sides of a semipermeable membrane if one side contains a nondiffusible or poorly diffusible ion. Let us first consider the situation illustrated in Figure 2-3, in which compart-

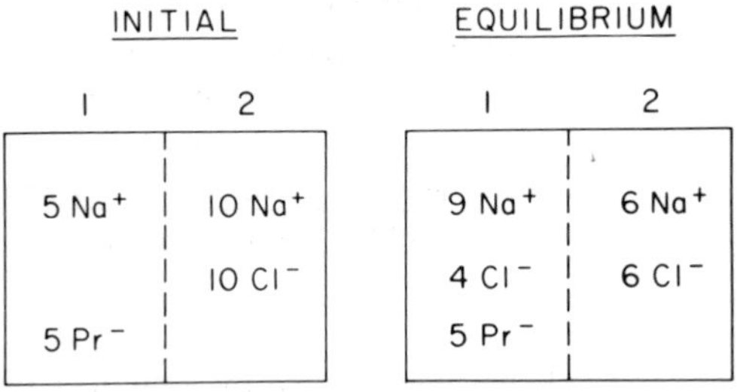

INITIAL

	1	2
	$5 Na^+$	$10 Na^+$
		$10 Cl^-$
	$5 Pr^-$	

EQUILIBRIUM

	1	2
	$9 Na^+$	$6 Na^+$
	$4 Cl^-$	$6 Cl^-$
	$5 Pr^-$	

Figure 2-3
The attainment of a Gibbs-Donnan equilibrium. Slightly modified from Pitts, R. F. *Physiology of the Kidney and Body Fluids,* 2d ed. Year Book, Chicago, 1968.

ments 1 and 2 are separated by a rigid membrane that is permeable to Na^+ and Cl^- but impermeable to protein, Pr^-. The rate at which either diffusible ion moves across the membrane will depend on the frequency with which it collides with the membrane, and that frequency is proportional to the concentration of the ion on each side of the membrane. Since the *difference* in concentration is initially greater for Cl^- than for Na^+, the rate of net movement of Cl^- from compartment 2 to compartment 1 will momentarily exceed that of Na^+. And since Pr^- cannot move across the membrane, a negative charge will be built up at the interface of the membrane. This electrostatic force will enhance the rate of net transfer of Na^+ from compartment 2 to compartment 1, so that in effect the rate of diffusion of both diffusible ions from compartment 2 to compartment 1 will be equal. Furthermore, this electrostatic force permits the buildup of Na^+ in compartment 1 against its concentration gradient, as the sytem approaches equilibrium. The work required to move one equivalent of Na^+ up its concentration gradient but down the electrical potential gradient is shown in Equation 2-3:

$$W = R \cdot T \cdot \log \frac{[Na^+]_1}{[Na^+]_2} - F \cdot E \qquad (2\text{-}3)$$

Where: $\quad$ W $\;=\;$ work

$\qquad\quad$ R $\;=\;$ gas constant

$\qquad\quad$ T $\;=\;$ absolute temperature

$[Na^+]_1$ and $[Na^+]_2$ $\;=\;$ concentrations of Na^+ in compartments 1 and 2, respectively

$\qquad\quad$ F $\;=\;$ Faraday

$\qquad\quad$ E $\;=\;$ electrical potential difference between the compartments.

The work required to move Cl^- down its concentration gradient but against the electrical potential gradient, will be

$$W = R \cdot T \cdot \log \frac{[Cl^-]_1}{[Cl^-]_2} + F \cdot E \qquad (2\text{-}4)$$

At equilibrium, by definition, no net work is performed by the system; hence, the sum of Equations 2-3 and 2-4 must be zero, and

$$\frac{[Na^+]_1}{[Na^+]_2} = \frac{[Cl^-]_2}{[Cl^-]_1} \qquad (2\text{-}5)$$

The equilibrium conditions of the Gibbs-Donnan effect can now be understood, and they are illustrated in Figure 2-3. (1) At equilibrium, the product of the concentrations of diffusible ions in one compartment will equal the product of the same ions in the other compartment (9 · 4 in compartment 1, and 6 · 6 in compartment 2). (2) Within each compartment the total cationic charges must equal the total anionic charges (9 of each in compartment 1; 6 in compartment 2). This requirement for electroneutrality is not in conflict with the existence of a small electrical P.D. across the membrane which, as noted earlier in this chapter, is confined to the interface and involves an insignificant fraction of the ions. (3) The concentration of diffusible cations will be greater in the compartment containing the nondiffusible, negatively charged protein than in the other compartment; and the concentration of diffusible anions will be less in compartment 1 than in compartment 2. (4) The osmolality will be greater in the compartment containing the protein (18 particles per equal volume) than in the other compartment (12 particles). The difference is due not only to the contained protein but also because the sum of the diffusible ions on the side containing the protein (9 + 4) is greater than the sum of these ions on the other side (6 + 6). The total difference in osmotic pressure that is due to the Gibbs-Donnan effect is known as the *oncotic pressure.*

These conditions hold also for the body fluid compartments, and apply to each of the diffusible ions within them. For example, each compartment is electrically neutral, and diffusible cations such as Na^+ are slightly more concentrated in plasma than in interstitial fluid, whereas the opposite is true of diffusible anions, such as Cl^- (Fig. 2-2). As has been noted, however, the osmolality of the intracellular compartment is actually the same as the interstitial osmolality, mainly because Na^+ is actively removed from cells.

Maintenance of Compartment Size

Importance of Total Solute Content

It follows from Equation 2-1 that for any given solute concentration, the volume or size of a compartment will be a direct function of the total amount of solute within it. The volumes of the main extracellular compartments, plasma and interstitium, depend primarily on the amount of Na^+ and its attendant anions (mainly Cl^- and HCO_3^-) in the body, since these constitute 90

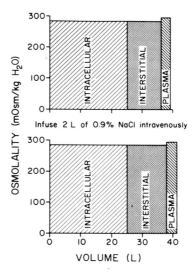

Figure 2-4

The effect of an intravenous infusion of NaCl having an osmolality of about 290 mOsm/kg H_2O on the volume and osmolal concentration of the body fluids. Note that there was no change in the osmolality of any compartment, and that the increase in volume involved only the plasma and interstitial compartments.

to 95% of the total osmotically active particles in extracellular fluid. Although by weight the plasma proteins have a high plasma concentration — about 70 g per liter — they contribute less than 1% to the total osmolality of plasma.

The effect of adding NaCl to the body is shown in Figure 2-4. Depicted at the top is the distribution of total body water in a healthy adult human, as it was summarized in Figure 2-1. A solution containing 0.9 g of NaCl per 100 ml of solution is then infused intravenously, i.e., into the plasma compartment; this solution has an osmolality of about 290 mOsm per kilogram H_2O. Since the capillary endothelium is highly permeable to Na^+, Cl^-, and H_2O, the infused solution is quickly distributed not only throughout the plasma, but also throughout the interstitial fluid. Although Na^+ will momentarily enter the intracellular space, it will be quickly "pumped out." Thus, there will be no gain or loss of Na^+ from the intracellular space, and since Cl^- follows Na^+, there will be no net change in Cl^-; that is, the solute and hence the H_2O that were added intravenously will be excluded from the intracellular space and will be distributed evenly throughout the extracellular compartment. Accordingly, to the extent that none of the added NaCl solution is lost from the body, the extracellular compartment will be expanded by 2 liters, and the infused solution will be distributed between plasma and inter-stitial fluid in proportion to their sizes prior to the infusion. Since the infused solution had about the same osmolality as the body fluids, there will be no change in the total solute concentration of extracellular fluid and hence no osmotic flow of water in or out of the intracellular compartment.

Maintenance of Plasma and Interstitial Volumes

The Starling Hypothesis. Because of the Gibbs-Donnan effect, the plasma has a slightly higher osmolality than does the interstitial fluid. Nevertheless, in the steady (equilibrium) state, the size of each compartment is stable. This is so mainly because the movement of water between the two compartments is governed by a balance between the oncotic pressure and the hydrostatic pressure within capillaries.

The forces that determine fluid exchange across the capillary endothelium were outlined by Starling in 1896. This formulation, known as the Starling hypothesis, is illustrated in Figure 2-5. The major force promoting filtration of fluid out of the capillary into the interstitium is the hydrostatic pressure within the capillaries. This pressure declines along the course of the capillary. A small amount of protein leaks out of the capillaries. Although most of this is returned to the systemic circulation via the lymph

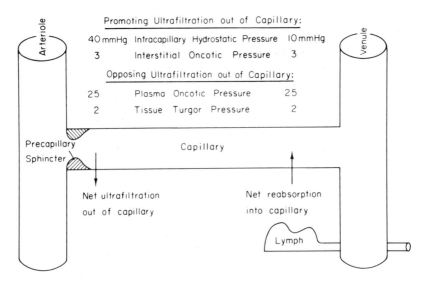

Figure 2-5
The Starling hypothesis of fluid exchange between plasma and interstitium. The four factors that determine this exchange are known as "Starling forces."

channels, some remains, giving rise to a small interstitial oncotic pressure of perhaps 3 mm Hg, which also promotes filtration out of the capillary. These two forces are opposed mainly by the plasma oncotic pressure and a small amount of pressure that is due to the turgidity of the interstitium. The balance of these forces is such that there is net filtration of fluid out of the capillary along slightly more than one-half of the length of the capillary, and net reabsorption of fluid into the capillary as it approaches the venule. The slight excess of fluid that is filtered into the interstitium is returned to the systemic plasma by the lymph channels, so that in the steady state the volumes of the two compartments, plasma and interstitium, remain constant.

Although the principle of opposing forces outlined in Figure 2-5 is correct, it seems likely that the main mechanism that ordinarily alters intracapillary hydrostatic pressure is not the resistance along the length of the capillary but rather the activity of the precapillary sphincters. When these relax, hydrostatic pressure throughout the capillary may be sufficiently high to promote net outward filtration along its entire length; when they contract, hydrostatic pressure may be so low that only reabsorption of fluid into the capillary occurs. Furthermore, the rate of fluid flow, $\dot{q}$, across the capillary endothelium, is a function not only of the Starling forces, but also of a filtration coefficient, K_f. Equation 2-6 expresses the total relationship:

$$\dot{q} = K_f \left[(P_c - P_t) - (\pi_p - \pi_t) \right] \tag{2-6}$$

where: $\dot{q}$ = rate of fluid movement across the capillary wall; K_f = the filtration coefficient; P_c = the intracapillary hydrostatic pressure; P_t = the tissue turgor pressure; π_p = the plasma oncotic pressure; and π_t = the interstitial oncotic pressure. The filtration coefficient is proportional to the total surface area of capillaries, as well as to capillary permeability per unit of surface area. When precapillary sphincters contract, many capillaries are actually shut off from the arterial circulation, so that total capillary surface area is reduced; relaxation of the sphincters during the vasodilator phase has the opposite effect. Thus, activity of the precapillary sphincters, so-called vasomotion, governs fluid flow across the capillary endothelium (Eq. 2-6) both by its effect on the intracapillary hydrostatic pressure, P_c, and on the filtration coefficient, K_f. The balance between the vasodilator and vasoconstrictor phases is such that the net return of fluid to plasma equals its net egress from this compartment (the return via the lymphatics making a very minor contribution).

Edema. Abnormal expansion of the interstitial fluid compartment, known as edema, is one of the most common findings in clinical medicine. According to Equation 2-6 one would predict increased $\dot{q}$, and hence appearance of edema, in a number of conditions that are in fact characterized by it: in inflammation because of a prolonged vasodilator phase; in congestive heart failure because an increased venous pressure raises intracapillary hydrostatic pressure; in liver failure because diminished synthesis of plasma proteins leads to decreased plasma oncotic pressure; in obstruction of lymphatic channels because failure to return proteins to the systemic circulation raises the interstitial oncotic pressure; and in old age because lower tissue elasticity decreases tissue turgor pressure.

Maintenance of Intracellular Volume

Why do cells that have a high oncotic pressure and are freely permeable to water not swell and burst? As noted earlier, the reason is that the distribution of Na^+ between the intracellular and interstitial compartments is not governed simply by the Gibbs-Donnan forces; rather, Na^+ is actively pumped out of cells. That this process requires metabolic energy is shown in Figure 2-6. When cells are deprived of such energy, as by exposing them to cold, or hypoxia, or metabolic inhibitors, they gain Na^+ and Cl^-, and with these solutes, water; that is, when the higher oncotic pressure of intracellular fluid is not opposed by the additional force of active Na^+ movement into the interstitium, cells do in fact swell and frequently burst. The fact that intracellular K^+ decreases when the cell is deprived of energy constitutes part of the evidence that the relatively high intracellular concentration of K^+ in control conditions is to some degree maintained by an active pump.

More than one-third of the metabolic energy of most cells is expended in transporting Na^+, thereby maintaining cellular volume. The question might well be asked why such an inefficient system has been invoked when the simpler expedient of a rigid, thick cellular membrane that excludes Na^+ from the cell interior might solve the problem as well. As was the case for general renal function (Chap. 1), so once again the answer probably lies in evolutionary selection, in this instance for a system that allowed great mobility, and that therefore required pliable cells with a large surface area to permit rapid diffusion of metabolic substrates.

Failure to prevent swelling of cells may be the cause of permanent ischemic damage, especially in the brain. Lack of

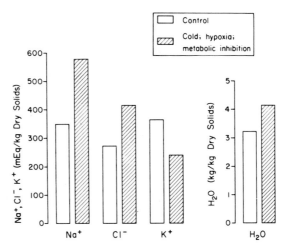

Figure 2-6
Effect of depriving cells of metabolic energy, on their content of Na^+, Cl^-, K^+, and H_2O. The heavy intracellular solutes did not change in this experiment. Hence, expressing the data per unit of dry weight makes it possible to interpret the results as content of the measured substances per approximately equal number of cells. Note that during metabolic inhibition, the loss of K^+ is less than the gains in Na^+ and Cl^-; this net entry of solute is followed by movement of H_2O into cells. The example is from cells of the renal cortex, which do not have the extremely low Na^+ and Cl^- concentrations and the high K^+ concentrations that skeletal muscle cells have (Fig. 2-2). But even in renal cortical cells, the concentrations of these ions differ greatly from those in extracellular fluid. Data from Leaf, A. *Amer. J. Med.* 49:291, 1970.

blood flow to the brain and, hence, lack of metabolic energy, lead to swelling not only of parenchymal cells but also of glial cells surrounding the microvasculature. The engorgement of glial cells may subsequently prevent capillary flow even though major blood flow to the affected area is quickly restored. This phenomenon, known as *no reflow*, may thus set up a chain of events in which swelling of a few critically situated perivascular glial cells leads to irreversible parenchymal damage.

Summary

Total body water, which comprises from 50 to 70% of the body weight, is distributed among three major compartments: (a) intracellular; (b) plasma; and (c) interstitial. The last two are the major subdivisions of extracellular fluid. Each compartment has a characteristic and stable size and composition. Sodium and its attendant anions are the major solutes in extracellular fluid. The main difference between plasma and interstitial fluid is the higher protein content in the former. The relative impermeability of the capillary endothelium to protein sets up a Gibbs-Donnan effect, which accounts for the slight differences in distribution of diffusible ions between plasma and interstitial fluid.

Organic phosphates and proteins are the major anions in most cells, and potassium is the main intracellular cation. The characteristic composition of intracellular fluid results from selective impermeabilities mainly for organic phosphates and proteins, the resulting Gibbs-Donnan equilibrium, binding to nondiffusible compounds, and active transport of sodium out of cells and potassium into them.

The volume of each compartment is fixed by the total solute within it. The steady size of the plasma and interstitial compartments is determined by the balance of Starling forces: (a) intracapillary hydrostatic pressure and (b) interstitial oncotic pressure favoring fluid movement out of the capillary; and (c) plasma oncotic pressure and (d) tissue turgor pressure favoring movement of fluid in the opposite direction.

Active "pumping" of sodium out of cells offsets the oncotic pressure of nondiffusible organic phosphates and proteins, and thereby ordinarily prevents swelling and bursting of cells.

Problem 2-1   *Note: The answers to this and subsequent problems are given in a special section at the end of the text.*

A woman weighing 60 kg is given 10 mg of T-1824 dye (Evans blue) intravenously. Ten minutes later, a blood sample is obtained from another vein, and colorimetric analysis of the plasma shows the presence of 0.4 mg of T-1824 per 100 ml of plasma.

Assume that the administered dye was evenly distributed throughout the plasma compartment by the end of the 10 minutes, and that no dye was lost from the plasma during this interval; then calculate the woman's plasma volume.

If the blood corpuscles, mainly erythrocytes, constituted 45% of whole blood — i.e., if the woman's hematocrit ratio is 0.45 — what is her total blood volume?

Problem 2-2   A man weighing 75 kg is given intravenously, 99.8 g of D_2O (i.e., 100 ml of a 99.8% solution of D_2O) and 100 μCi of radiosulfate (^{35}S-sulfate). Twenty minutes after injection, a blood sample is drawn and treated to obtain a protein-free filtrate of plasma. A second blood sample is drawn 2 hours after the injection, and similarly treated. Exactly 1 ml of the first filtrate is found to contain 0.0064 μCi of radiosulfate. The water of the second filtrate is found to contain 0.2 g D_2O per 100 ml of filtrate.

Assume: (a) that 4% of the injected radiosulfate was lost in the urine during the first 20 minutes; (b) that 0.4% of the administered D_2O was lost during the 2 hours; (c) that no other losses of these two substances occurred; and (d) that radiosulfate and D_2O were evenly distributed throughout their compartments after 20 minutes and 2 hours, respectively.

Calculate: (a) total body water, (b) extracellular fluid volume, and (c) intracellular fluid volume.

Selected References

General

Bernard, C. *Leçons sur les Phénomèns de la Vie Communs aux Animaux et aux Végétaux,* vol. I. Baillière, Paris, 1878.

Dick, D. A. T. *Cell Water.* Butterworth, Washington, 1966.

Edelman, I. S., and Leibman, J. Anatomy of body water and electrolytes. *Amer. J. Med.* 27:256, 1959.

Elkinton, J. R., and Danowski, T. S. *The Body Fluids.* Williams & Wilkins, Baltimore, 1955.

Gamble, J. L. *Chemical Anatomy, Physiology and Pathology of Extracellular Fluid,* 6th ed. Harvard University Press, Cambridge, 1954.

Lockwood, A. P. M. *Animal Body Fluids and Their Regulation.* Harvard University Press, Cambridge, 1966.

Manery, J. F. Water and electrolyte metabolism. *Physiol. Rev.* 34:334, 1954.

Maxwell, M. H., and Kleeman, C. R. (Eds.). *Clinical Disorders of Fluid and Electrolyte Metabolism,* 2d ed. McGraw-Hill, New York, 1972.

Moore, F. D. *Metabolic Care of the Surgical Patient.* Saunders, Philadelphia, 1959.

Peters, J. P. *Body Water: The Exchange of Fluids in Man.* Thomas, Springfield, Ill., 1935.

Robinson, J. R. Metabolism of intracellular water. *Physiol. Rev.* 40:112, 1960.

Strauss, M. B. *Body Water in Man: The Acquisition and Maintenance of the Body Fluids.* Little, Brown, Boston, 1957.

Welt, L. G. *Clinical Disorders of Hydration and Acid-Base Equilibrium,* 2d ed. Little, Brown, Boston, 1959.

Widdowson, E. M., McCance, R. A., and Spray, C. M. The chemical composition of the human body. *Clin. Sci.* 10:113, 1951.

Evolution   Macallum, A. B. The paleochemistry of the body fluids and tissues. *Physiol. Rev.* 6:316, 1926.
Robertson, J. D. The habitat of the early vertebrates. *Biol. Rev.* 32:156, 1957.

Gibbs-Donnan   Spiegler, K. S., and Wyllie, M. R. J. Electrical Potential Differences. In G. Oster and A. W. Pollister (Eds.), *Physical Techniques in Biological Research,* vol. II. Academic, New York, 1956.
West, E. S., Todd, W. R., Mason, H. S., and van Bruggen, J. T. *Textbook of Biochemistry,* 4th ed. Macmillan, New York, 1966.

Measurement of   Brown, E., Hopper, J., Jr., Hodges, J. L., Jr., Bradley, B.,
Compartment   Wennesland, R., and Yamauchi, H. Red cell, plasma, and
Size   blood volume in healthy women measured by radio-chromium cell-labeling and hematocrit. *J. Clin. Invest.* 41:2182, 1962.
Deane, N. Methods of Study of Body Water Compartments. In A. C. Corcoran (Ed.), *Methods in Medical Research,* vol. V. Year Book, Chicago, 1952.
Gaudino, M., and Levitt, M. F. Inulin space as a measure of extracellular fluid. *Amer. J. Physiol.* 157:387, 1949.
Moore, F. D., Olesen, K. H., McMurrey, J. D., Parker, H. V., Ball, M. R., and Boyden, C. M. *The Body Cell Mass and Its Supporting Environment. Body Composition in Health and Disease.* Saunders, Philadelphia, 1963.
Schloerb, P. R., Friis-Hansen, B. J., Edelman, I. S., Solomon, A. K., and Moore, F. D. The measurement of total body water in the human subject by deuterium oxide dilution. *J. Clin. Invest.* 29:1296, 1950.
Schultz, A. L., Hammarsten, J. F., Heller, B. I., and Ebert, R. V. A critical comparison of the T-1824 dye and iodinated albumin methods for plasma volume measurement. *J. Clin. Invest.* 32:107, 1953.
Sterling, K., and Gray, S. J. Determination of the circulating red cell volume in man by radioactive chromium. *J. Clin. Invest.* 29:1614, 1950.

Walser, M., Seldin, D. W., and Grollman, A. An evaluation of radiosulfate for the determination of the volume of extracellular fluid in man and dogs. *J. Clin. Invest.* 32:299, 1953.

Regulation of
Compartment
Size

Ames, A., III, Wright, L., Kowada, M., Thurston, J. M., and Majno, G. Cerebral ischemia: II. The no-reflow phenomenon. *Amer. J. Pathol.* 52:437, 1968.

Appleboom, J. W. T., Brodsky, W. A., Tuttle, W. S., and Diamond, I. The freezing point depression of mammalian tissues after sudden heating in boiling distilled water. *J. Gen. Physiol.* 41:1153, 1958.

Flores, J., diBona, D. R., Beck, C. H., and Leaf, A. The role of cell swelling in ischemic renal damage and the protective effect of hypertonic solute. *J. Clin. Invest.* 51:118, 1972.

Krogh, A. *Osmotic Regulation in Aquatic Animals.* University Press, Cambridge, 1939. (Reprinted unabridged and unaltered by Dover Publications, New York, 1965.)

Landis, E. M. *The Passage of Fluid Through the Capillary Wall.* The Harvey Lectures, Series XXXII. Williams & Wilkins, Baltimore, 1937.

Leaf, A. Regulation of intracellular fluid volume and disease. *Amer. J. Med.* 49:291, 1970.

Maffly, R. H., and Leaf, A. The potential of water in mammalian tissues. *J. Gen. Physiol.* 42:1257, 1959.

Mudge, G. H. Studies on potassium accumulation by rabbit kidney slices: Effect of metabolic activity. *Amer. J. Physiol.* 165:113, 1951.

Pappenheimer, J. R. Passage of molecules through capillary walls. *Physiol. Rev.* 33:387, 1953.

Starling, E. H. On the absorption of fluids from the connective tissue spaces. *J. Physiol.* 19:312, 1896.

Starling, E. H. *The Fluids of the Body.* Keener, Chicago, 1909.

Zweifach, B. W. *Functional Behavior of the Microcirculation.* Thomas, Springfield, Ill., 1961.

3 : Glomerular Filtration

Ultrafiltration

This process occurs at the glomeruli and is filtration under pressure through the permselective glomerular capillary wall. Ultrafiltration separates the plasma water and its nonprotein constituents (often referred to as crystalloids), which enter Bowman's space, from the blood cells and protein macromolecules (the colloids), which stay in the blood. The process is thus qualitatively the same as that occurring in systemic capillaries, although, as we shall see, the two are quantitatively different.

Proof for ultrafiltration by glomeruli was first obtained in 1921 by J. T. Wearn and A. N. Richards, through the technique of micropuncture. They succeeded in collecting fluid from Bowman's space by means of a tiny micropipet having a tip diameter of 7 to 15 μm. The collected fluid contained no protein as measured by methods then available (actually, small amounts of protein are filtered and then reabsorbed), and it had approximately the same composition as plasma in respect to osmolality, electrical conductivity (i.e., total concentration of electrolytes), glucose and other solutes, and pH. Furthermore, the distribution of diffusible electrolytes between glomerular capillary plasma and fluid in Bowman's space conformed to the Gibbs-Donnan relationship. The early results were obtained in amphibians, the frog and *Necturus,* and they have since been confirmed in rodents, dogs, primates, and other species.

Forces Involved in Glomerular Ultrafiltration

These are the so-called Starling forces which were reviewed for systemic capillaries in Chapter 2 and Figure 2-5. Those pertaining to mammalian glomeruli are shown in Figure 3-1. There are several differences. (1) Hydrostatic pressure remains relatively constant in glomerular capillaries, whereas it declines markedly along the length of extrarenal capillaries. (2) Glomerular capillaries are probably less permeable to proteins than systemic capillaries. Hence, the oncotic pressure in Bow-

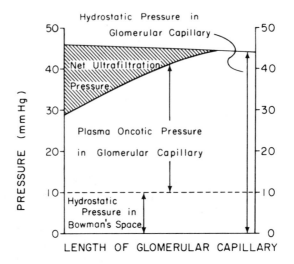

BALANCE OF MEAN VALUES

Hydrostatic pressure in glomerular capillary	45 mmHg
Hydrostatic pressure in Bowman's space	10
Plasma oncotic pressure in glomerular capillary	27
Oncotic pressure of fluid in Bowman's space	0
Net ultrafiltration pressure	8 mmHg

Figure 3-1
Forces involved in glomerular ultrafiltration in rats. As shown, ultrafiltration pressure declines in glomerular capillaries, mainly because plasma oncotic pressure rises. This is in contrast to extrarenal capillaries, in which the decline in ultrafiltration pressure is due mainly to a decrease in intracapillary hydrostatic pressure (see Fig. 2-5). The pattern for the rise in plasma oncotic pressure as a function of capillary length is not known precisely; hence, the mean values for plasma oncotic and net ultra-filtration pressures listed in the table are approximations. It is not yet known at what point in the capillary the sum of the hydrostatic pressure in Bowman's space and of plasma oncotic pressure exactly balances the hydrostatic pressure in the glomerular capillary. If, as shown here, this occurs before the end of the capillary is reached, ultrafiltration would not take place over the entire length of the glomerular capillary. Data from Brenner, B. M., Troy, J. L., and Daugharty, T. M. *J. Clin. Invest.* 50:1776, 1971.

man's space is lower than interstitial oncotic pressure. (3) In contrast to the plasma oncotic pressure in systemic capillaries, which stays relatively constant, that in glomerular capillaries rises along the length of the capillary. (4) The hydrostatic pressure in Bowman's space is considerably higher than its systemic analogue, the tissue turgor pressure. Nevertheless, the balance of the forces is such that the mean net ultrafiltration pressure in glomerular capillaries is similar to that existing at the arteriolar end of extrarenal capillaries. In the latter (Fig. 2-5), net ultrafiltration pressure declines because capillary hydrostatic pressure decreases, whereas in glomerular capillaries, net ultrafiltration pressure declines mainly because plasma oncotic pressure increases. Furthermore, in glomerular capillaries, net movement of fluid is primarily out of the capillaries, whereas in systemic capillaries the change in the balance of Starling forces is such that net movement out of the vessels is nearly balanced by net return of fluid into the vessels.

Even though the mean net ultrafiltration pressures are similar in glomerular and extrarenal capillaries, the transtubular movement of fluid out of glomerular capillaries, the so-called glomerular filtration rate (GFR), far exceeds the analogous flow, $\dot{q}$ of Equation 2-6, in extrarenal capillaries. Hence K_f, the filtration coefficient, must be much larger for glomerular capillaries. This conclusion suggests that the glomerular capillary differs from other capillaries, for example, from those of skeletal muscle. We shall therefore next consider some of the distinctions.

Characteristics of the Glomerular Capillary

As defined in Chapter 2, K_f is a function of total capillary surface area as well as of the permeability per unit of surface area. Both factors are probably involved in raising the K_f of glomerular capillaries. Total glomerular capillary area has been estimated to be from 5,000 to 15,000 cm^2 per 100 g of renal tissue. In contrast, this area is perhaps 7,000 cm^2 per 100 g of skeletal muscle. In addition, per unit of surface area, glomerular capillaries may be at least 100 times more permeable to water and crystalloids than muscle capillaries.

Both glomerular and extrarenal capillaries permit free passage of small molecules such as water (2 Å diameter), urea (3.2 Å diameter), sodium (4 Å diameter), chloride (3.5 Å diameter), and glucose (7 Å diameter); but they do not permit free passage of larger particles such as erythrocytes (80,000 Å diameter) or large plasma proteins. The limits of glomerular capillary permeability are suggested by the fact that hemoglobin (65 Å diameter), as well as smaller plasma proteins such as albumin (36 by 150 Å), are not freely filtered but do get through the membrane in small amounts. In other words, the glomerular capillary behaves as if it were a filtering membrane containing aqueous "pores" with a diameter of 75 to 100 Å.

Given these functional characteristics, anatomists have examined the wall of the glomerular capillary, to see if it contained a structure with fenestrations of the required dimensions. The wall (Fig. 3-2c) consists of three layers: (a) endothe-

(a)　　　　　　Capillary Loops　　　　　　　　　Bowman's Space

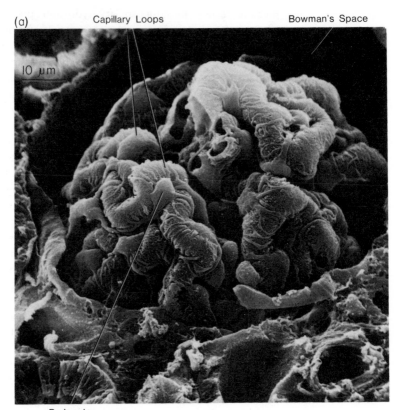

10 μm

Podocyte

Figure 3-2
Electron scan photomicrographs of: (a) a glomerulus, magnified about
1,440 times; and (b) a loop of a glomerular capillary, magnified about
7,200 times. An electron micrograph (X 36,000) of a glomerular capillary,
viewed in longitudinal section, is shown in (c). Photomicrographs (a) and
(b) from: Spinelli, F., Wirz, H., and Brücher, C. *Fine Structure of the
Kidney Revealed by Scanning Electron-Microscopy.* Ciba-Geigy, Basle,
1972. The electron micrograph (c) was kindly supplied by C. C. Tisher.

(b) Podocyte

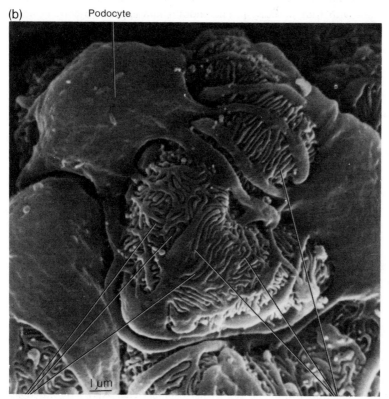

1 μm

Filtration Slits   Foot Processes

0.3 μm

Bowman's Space

(c)

Foot Processes

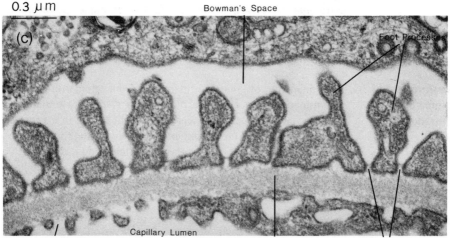

Pore in Endothelium   Capillary Lumen   Basement Membrane   Filtration Slits

lium, (b) basement membrane, and (c) epithelium (podocytes with foot processes). The endothelium appears to contain holes with a diameter of 500 to 1,000 Å. Most investigators believe that these apertures, unlike those of other fenestrated capillaries, are not bridged by diaphragms. The glomerular endothelium, therefore, appears to be freely permeable even to large molecules. The basement membrane is a continuous, filamentous layer that is fused with both the endothelium and the epithelium. Some believe this to be the restrictive layer. The epithelium consists of highly specialized cells called podocytes, which are attached to the basement membrane by foot processes known as pedicels. Adjacent pedicels are separated by filtration slits measuring about 250 Å in width, and each gap may be bridged by a thin diaphragm. Experiments with two proteins of different dimensions suggest that these slits with their diaphragms may be the semipermeable filtration barrier. Horseradish peroxidase, having a molecular weight of about 40,000 and a diameter of about 50 Å, passes readily through all three layers of the glomerular capillary wall into Bowman's space. In contrast, myeloperoxidase (molecular weight of about 170,000 and diameter of about 80 Å) passes quickly through the endothelium and basement membrane, but is held up at the filtration slits.

Actually, anatomical pores as such may not exist. The functional characteristics of glomerular capillaries could be accounted for as well if the restrictive barrier, whatever its location within the glomerular capillary wall, were a hydrated gel without permanent channels. What does seem clear is that the higher transmural filtration rate of glomerular as opposed to extrarenal capillaries, is due both to a much higher permeability to water and crystalloids per unit of surface area and to a larger capillary surface area per unit of tissue.

Measurement of Glomerular Filtration Rate (GFR)

The quantity of plasma filtered by the glomeruli can be determined by the clearance of inulin, a starch-like polymer of fructose having a molecular weight of about 5,000. It is a foreign substance and must be infused intravenously during the clearance test. Since it is not bound to plasma proteins and has a diameter of about 30 Å, it passes readily through the glomerular capillary membrane. In addition, it is neither reabsorbed nor secreted by renal tubules.

In Figure 3-3, both kidneys of a normal adult man are represented by a single nephron. The principle for measuring GFR by the clearance technique is illustrated by the following steps.

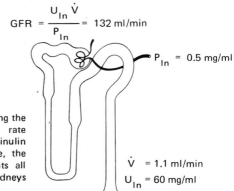

$$\text{GFR} = \frac{U_{In} \dot{V}}{P_{In}} = 132 \text{ ml/min}$$

$P_{In} = 0.5 \text{ mg/ml}$

$\dot{V} = 1.1 \text{ ml/min}$

$U_{In} = 60 \text{ mg/ml}$

Figure 3-3
The principle of measuring the glomerular filtration rate (GFR) by means of the inulin clearance. In this figure, the single nephron represents all nephrons from both kidneys of adult man.

1. Measure the rate of urine flow, $\dot{V}$; $\dot{V}$ = 1.1 ml/min.
2. Measure the concentration of inulin in the urine, U_{In}; U_{In} = 60 mg/ml.
3. Calculate the amount of inulin excreted in the urine per minute.

$$U_{In} \cdot \dot{V} = \frac{60 \text{ mg}}{\text{ml}} \cdot \frac{1.1 \text{ ml}}{\text{min}} = 66 \text{ mg/min}$$

4. If: (a) all inulin reaching the urine got there by filtration, and
   (b) inulin was not reabsorbed from the tubular lumen, and
   (c) inulin was not secreted into the tubular lumen, and
   (d) the plasma concentration of inulin, P_{In}, was 0.5 mg/ml; i.e., if each milliliter of plasma contained 0.5 mg of inulin, how many milliliters of plasma must have been filtered in order to excrete 66 mg of inulin?

$$66 \text{ mg} \div \frac{0.5 \text{ mg}}{\text{ml}} = 132 \text{ ml}$$

5. Since 66 mg of inulin was excreted per minute, 132 ml of plasma must have been filtered each minute.

$$\frac{66 \text{ mg}}{\text{min}} \div \frac{0.5 \text{ mg}}{\text{ml}} = \frac{66 \text{ mg}}{\text{min}} \cdot \frac{\text{ml}}{0.5 \text{ mg}} = 132 \text{ ml/min}$$

Thus, during each minute, 132 ml of plasma was separated by ultrafiltration from the blood flowing through the glomerular capillaries. This measurement is called the *inulin clearance,* C_{In}. It is defined as the volume of plasma from which, in a minute's time, the kidneys remove all inulin.

Several features of this measurement should be noted. (a) The equation for all renal clearances is $U \cdot \dot{V}/P$, where U is the concentration of a given substance in the urine, $\dot{V}$ is the urine flow, and P is the concentration of the same substance in the plasma. *The clearance technique is not confined to the measurement of GFR;* it can and is applied to many substances besides inulin. (b) *Plasma,* not urine, is being cleared of a given substance, in this case inulin. The units for the inulin clearance refer to the milliliters of *plasma* from which all inulin has been removed. (c) The inulin clearance is independent of the plasma inulin concentration; as P_{In} increases, more inulin will be filtered so that U_{In} will rise in direct proportion to the increase in P_{In} (Fig. 3-3). (d) The inulin clearance is independent of the urine flow; for a given quantity of inulin in the urine, U_{In} will fall proportionately as $\dot{V}$ rises, and vice versa. Points (c) and (d) are illustrated in Problem 3-1, at the end of this chapter.

Concept of
Filtration
Fraction

Not all the plasma that flows through the glomerular capillaries can be filtered into Bowman's space. This would be an obvious impossibility, for it would require the transmural movement of all plasma, leaving behind a solid mass of cells and colloids that could not move on into the efferent arterioles. As is shown in Figure 3-1, long before this state is reached, filtration stops because the sum of the hydrostatic pressure in Bowman's space plus the rising plasma oncotic pressure equals the hydrostatic pressure in the glomerular capillaries. Normally, only about one-fifth of the plasma entering the glomerular capillaries is filtered; this is called the *filtration fraction,* the definition and derivation of which are given in Chapter 5.

Inulin: Neither Reabsorbed nor Secreted. Use of the inulin clearance as a measure of GFR is valid only if all the inulin that appears in the urine got there by filtration, i.e., only if inulin is neither reabsorbed nor secreted by the renal tubules. Proof that these conditions are met was obtained through a number of micropuncture experiments, one of which is shown in Figure 3-4. A proximal tubule of a rat was punctured at E from the surface of the kidney, and a column of oil, C, was injected via a micropipet in order to block the tubular lumen. This pipet was then withdrawn, leaving an opening at E through which newly formed glomerular filtrate could escape. A second pipet, A, was then inserted distal to the oil column, and a green dye was

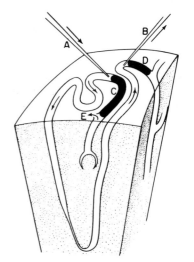

Figure 3-4
A micropuncture experiment in a rat kidney. The symbols, as well as the rationale of the experiment, are explained in the text. The arrows indicate the direction of flow of tubular fluid. From Marsh, D., and Frasier, C. *Amer. J. Physiol.* 209:283, 1965. Published with permission.

injected. This dye traversed the remainder of the proximal tubule and the loop of Henle, and reappeared on the surface of the kidney in the distal tubule belonging to this single nephron. A third pipet, B, was then inserted into the distal segment, and the remainder of the tubule was blocked with a second oil column, D.

A known amount of inulin was now infused into the proximal segment through pipet A at the same time that all fluid perfusing that nephron was collected through pipet B. The fact that 99.3% of the injected inulin could be thus recovered strongly suggests that inulin was not reabsorbed. Furthermore, the rate of recovery was the same when the peritubular plasma was loaded with inulin; hence secretion of inulin was also excluded. Finally when oil block D was not present, virtually all the inulin microinjected into the proximal tubule could be recovered in the ureteral urine. Thus, inulin is neither reabsorbed nor secreted in any portion of the nephron.

Other Substances. There are substances besides inulin that are also freely filtered but neither reabsorbed nor secreted by the renal tubules. Hence such substances, too, can be used to measure GFR. Some substances meet the criteria in one species but not in others. For example, under physiological conditions, creatinine is neither reabsorbed nor secreted in the dog, and is therefore equal to the inulin clearance. In man, however, the creatinine clearance is slightly higher than the GFR because the renal tubules secrete a small amount of creatinine. The identity of the inulin and creatinine clearances in a dog under physiological conditions are illustrated by the calculations given in Problem 3-2 at the end of this chapter.

Clearance as a General Concept

It was emphasized above that the clearance concept is not restricted to the determination of GFR. One can measure the renal clearance of any substance, and the comparison of that clearance to that of inulin has important functional implications. For example, if, during any given time interval, less plasma is cleared of urea (a small molecule which is freely filterable) than is cleared of inulin, one can deduce that there must have been net reabsorption of urea in its course through the tubular system. (A quantitative example of this deduction is given in the Answers to Problems 4-1 and 8-1 at the end of the text.) Conversely, if during a given time interval, more plasma is cleared of a substance than is cleared of inulin, that substance must have been added to the urine by an additional process besides glomerular filtration; that process, called tubular secretion, is discussed in Chapter 5.

Finally, it should be stressed that the clearance concept is by no means restricted to renal function. One can measure the rates at which the lungs, or the liver, or other organs clear plasma of a given substance; or one can determine the so-called total, or "whole-body," clearance, which represents the sum of the various regional clearances. Such applications of the clearance concept are commonly applied to the study of drug or hormone metabolism.

Significance of TF/P and U/P for Inulin

Not only is inulin freely filtered, it is also a nonelectrolyte and therefore not subject to a Gibbs-Donnan effect. Hence, the concentration of inulin in Bowman's capsule fluid (TF_{In} = inulin concentration in tubular fluid) will be identical to that in plasma, P_{In}. The ratio of the concentration of inulin in Bowman's capsule fluid to that in plasma, referred to as the TF/P inulin, will therefore equal 1. Since inulin is neither reabsorbed from nor secreted into the tubular lumen, its concentration in tubular fluid increases as water is reabsorbed from the various tubular segments; in fact, the concentration of inulin in the tubular fluid will be solely a function of the amount of water reabsorbed up to the point at which the tubule is punctured and a microsample is withdrawn.

For example, if the concentration of inulin in tubular fluid withdrawn from the proximal tubule is twice as great as that in Bowman's space (i.e., in plasma), it is obvious that 50% of the filtered water must have been reabsorbed. Hence, a TF/P inulin of 2 reflects reabsorption of one-half of the filtered water, and the formula for calculating this fraction is given in Equation 3-1:

$$\text{Fraction of filtered water reabsorbed up to point of micropuncture} = 1 - \frac{1}{\text{TF/P inulin}}$$

$$= 1 - \frac{1}{2} \qquad (3\text{-}1)$$

$$= 0.5, \text{ or } 50\%.$$

Micropuncture samples withdrawn from the very last segment of a proximal tubule at the surface of the kidney usually have inulin concentrations that are nearly 3 times greater than the concentration in plasma; that is, TF/P inulin = 3, and the fraction of filtered water reabsorbed = 0.67. This, in fact, constitutes some of the experimental evidence that roughly two-thirds, or 67%, of the filtered fluid is normally reabsorbed in the proximal tubule.

By similar reasoning, the U/P inulin (the ratio of the concentration of inulin in the urine to its concentration in plasma) can be used to calculate the fraction of filtrate reabsorbed in both kidneys, as given in Equation 3-2:

$$\text{Fraction of filtered water reabsorbed by both kidneys} = 1 - \frac{1}{\text{U/P inulin}} \qquad (3\text{-}2)$$

In the example given in Figure 3-3, $1 - \frac{1}{120} = 0.992$; i.e., 99.2% of the filtered water was reabsorbed. (This point can be verified independently by calculating that the urine flow of 1.1 ml/min constitutes 0.8% of the amount of fluid filtered, 132 ml/min.)

Summary

The initial step in the formation of urine is ultrafiltration of plasma in the glomerular capillaries. As in other capillaries, the rate of this process is governed by: (a) Starling forces; (b) the permeability of the glomerular capillary wall to water and small solutes; and (c) the total surface area of the capillaries. The last two factors are greater in glomerular than in most extrarenal capillaries; hence, the rate of glomerular filtration (GFR) far exceeds analogous movement of fluid across walls of most systemic capillaries.

The GFR can be measured by the inulin clearance, which is defined as the volume of plasma from which, in a minute's time, the kidneys remove all inulin. Normally, about one-fifth of the plasma that flows through the glomerular capillaries is filtered into Bowman's space.

Since inulin, once filtered, is neither reabsorbed from nor secreted into the tubular lumen, the degree to which it is concentrated in tubular fluid will be solely a function of the amount of filtered water that is reabsorbed. Normally, about 70% of the filtered water is reabsorbed in the proximal tubules, and more than 99% is reabsorbed by the entire tubular system of both kidneys.

Problem 3-1. Sample calculations illustrating the independence of the inulin clearance from the plasma concentration of inulin and from the rate of urine flow in a dog. Utilizing the data given, calculate the inulin clearances. The answers are given at the end of the text.

| Urine Flow (ml/min) | Inulin Concentration | | Inulin Clearance (ml/min) |
	Plasma (mg/ml)	Urine (mg/ml)	
1.3	0.5	24	
1.2	0.9	45	
1.3	1.4	68	
1.0	2.3	141	
1.4	3.8	168	
1.2	5.7	294	
1.3	0.5	23	
1.7	0.6	22	
2.1	0.6	17	
3.1	0.4	8	
5.7	0.5	5	
6.6	0.5	4.6	

Modified from Shannon, J. A. *Amer. J. Physiol.* 112:405, 1935.

Problem 3-2. Sample calculations illustrating the identity of the inulin and creatinine clearances in a dog under physiological conditions. Utilizing the data given, calculate the inulin and creatinine clearances.

Urine Flow (ml/min)	Inulin			Creatinine		
	Plasma (mg/100 ml)	Urine (mg/100 ml)	Clearance (ml/min)	Plasma (mg/100 ml)	Urine (mg/100 ml)	Clearance (ml/min)
1.0	104	5,076		13.7	673	
1.1	106	4,601		14.7	630	
0.9	108	6,017		16.0	890	
1.0	109	5,137		16.6	792	

Modified from Shannon, J. A. *Amer. J. Physiol. 112:405, 1935.*

Selected References

The Process of Ultrafiltration

Pappenheimer, J. R. Passage of molecules through capillary walls. *Physiol. Rev.* 33:387, 1953.

Pappenheimer, J. R., Renkin, E. M., and Borrero, L. M. Filtration, diffusion and molecular sieving through peripheral capillary membranes: A contribution to the pore theory of capillary permeability. *Amer. J. Physiol.* 167:13, 1951.

Richards, A. N. *Urine Formation in the Amphibian Kidney.* The Harvey Lectures, Series XXX, 1934–35. Williams & Wilkins, Baltimore, 1936.

Walker, A., Bott, P., Oliver, J., and MacDowell, M. The collection and analysis of fluid from single nephrons of the mammalian kidney. *Amer. J. Physiol.* 134:580, 1941.

Wearn, J. T., and Richards, A. N. Observations on the composition of glomerular urine, with particular reference to the problem of reabsorption in the renal tubules. *Amer. J. Physiol.* 71:209, 1924.

Forces Determining Glomerular Ultrafiltration

Brenner, B. M., Troy, J. L., and Daugharty, T. M. The dynamics of glomerular ultrafiltration in the rat. *J. Clin. Invest.* 50:1776, 1971.

Renkin, E. M., and Gilmore, J. Glomerular Filtration. In J. Orloff and R. W. Berliner (Eds.), *Handbook of Physiology.* Section 8: Renal Physiology. American Physiological Society, Washington, D.C., 1973.

Measurement of GFR

Austin, J. H., Stillman, E., and van Slyke, D. D. Factors governing the excretion rate of urea. *J. Biol. Chem.* 46:91, 1921.

Gutman, Y., Gottschalk, C. W., and Lassiter, W. E. Micropuncture study of inulin absorption in the rat. *Science* 147:753, 1965.

Jolliffe, N., Shannon, J. A., and Smith, H. W. The excretion of urine in the dog: III. The use of non-metabolized sugars in the measurement of the glomerular filtrate. *Amer. J. Physiol.* 100:301, 1932.

Marsh, D., and Frasier, C. Reliability of inulin for measuring volume flow in rat renal cortical tubules. *Amer. J. Physiol.* 209:283, 1965.

Mertz, D. P., and Sarre, H. Polyfructosan-S:Eine neue inulin-artige Substanz zur Bestimmung des Glomerulusfiltrates und des physiologisch aktiven extrazellulären Flüssigkeits-volumens beim Menschen. *Klin. Wschr.* 41:868, 1963.

Nelps, W. B., Wagner, H. N., Jr., and Reba, R. C. Renal excretion of vitamin B_{12} and its use in measurement of glomerular filtration rate in man. *J. Lab. Clin. Med.* 63:480, 1964.

O'Connell, J. M. B., Romeo, J. A., and Mudge, G. H. Renal tubular secretion of creatinine in the dog. *Amer. J. Physiol.* 203:985, 1962.

Rehberg, P. B. Studies on kidney function: I. The rate of filtration and reabsorption in the human kidney. *Biochem. J.* 20:447, 1926.

Shannon, J. A. The excretion of inulin by the dog. *Amer. J. Physiol.* 112:405, 1935.

Tanner, G. A., and Klose, R. M. Micropuncture study of inulin reabsorption in *Necturus* kidney. *Amer. J. Physiol.* 211:1036, 1966.

Wright, F. S., and Giebisch, G. Glomerular filtration in single nephrons. *Kidney Int.* 1:201, 1972.

Clearance Concept

Austin, J. H., Stillman, E., and van Slyke, D. D. Factors governing the excretion rate of urea. *J. Biol. Chem.* 46:91, 1921.

Lauson, H. D. Metabolism of antidiuretic hormones. *Amer. J. Med.* 42:713, 1967.

Smith, H. W. *The Kidney: Structure and Function in Health and Disease.* Oxford University Press, New York, 1951.

Characteristics of Glomerular Capillaries

Latta, H. The glomerular capillary wall. *J. Ultrastruct. Res.* 32:526, 1970.

Venkatachalam, M. A., Karnovsky, M. J., and Cotran, R. S. Glomerular permeability: Ultrastructural studies in experimental nephrosis using horseradish peroxidase as a tracer. *J. Exper. Med.* 130:381, 1969.

Venkatachalam, M. A., Karnovsky, M. J., Fahimi, H. D., and Cotran, R. S. An ultrastructural study of glomerular permeability using catalase and peroxidase as tracer proteins. *J. Exper. Med.* 132:1153, 1970.

4 : Tubular Reabsorption

Water and many solutes are reabsorbed from the tubular lumen into the peritubular interstitial fluid and thence into the blood. Since the activities of water and small molecules in interstitial fluid are virtually identical to those in plasma, we often speak of reabsorption directly into the blood. The term *reabsorption* refers to the *direction* of transport, i.e., out of the tubular lumen; it may be applied to all modes of transport in that direction, be they active or passive.

Generally speaking, tubular reabsorption facilitates the conservation of substances that are essential to normal function — e.g., water, glucose and other sugars, amino acids, and electrolytes. Many of these substances, such as glucose and amino acids, are reabsorbed primarily or exclusively by the proximal tubules, whereas others, such as water and sodium, are also reabsorbed at more distal sites in the nephron.

Qualitative Evidence for Reabsorption

The most obvious examples are water, and Na^+ with its main accompanying anions, Cl^- and HCO_3^-. For these substances, which are considered in subsequent chapters, more than 99% of the loads that are filtered are reabsorbed (see Table 1-1). In this chapter, however, we shall concentrate on the reabsorption of solutes other than sodium and its attendant anions. Glucose is a simple case in point. This sugar, having a molecular diameter of about 7 Å and not being bound to plasma proteins, is freely filtered through the glomerular capillary wall and appears in Bowman's space fluid at the same concentration as in plasma. The fact that normally almost no glucose appears in the urine therefore shows that the sugar must be reabsorbed. Micropuncture studies have shown that about 99% of the filtered glucose is reabsorbed in the proximal tubule, nearly all of this in the first half of the proximal tubule. Furthermore, since the plasma concentration of glucose is much higher than that in urine, glucose must be reabsorbed against a concentration gradient, i.e., its reabsorption must be at least in part active.

Reabsorption of glucose can be blocked by a glucoside, phlorizin. When this compound is given to an animal, glucose appears in the urine, and the U/P ratio for glucose (i.e., the ratio of the concentration of glucose in urine to that in plasma) is identical to the U/P ratio for inulin. As reviewed in Chapter 3, the U/P ratio for inulin is a function solely of water reabsorption. Hence, the identity of the two ratios during administration of phlorizin must mean that all glucose reabsorption was blocked so that urinary glucose was concentrated by water reabsorption, to the same extent as inulin.

Quantifying Reabsorption

Net reabsorption for all nephrons combined can be measured using the following formula:

$$\text{Quantity excreted} = \text{quantity filtered} - \text{quantity reabsorbed} \qquad (4\text{-}1)$$

For inorganic phosphate, an electrolyte that is actively re-absorbed — i.e., reabsorbed against an electrochemical potential gradient at the expense of energy derived from metabolism:

$$\text{Quantity excreted} = U_P \cdot \dot{V}$$

$$\text{Quantity filtered} = P_P \cdot \text{GFR}$$

where U_P = the concentration of phosphate in urine; $\dot{V}$ = the rate of urine flow; P_P = the concentration of inorganic phosphate in plasma; and GFR = the glomerular filtration rate. If GFR is determined by the clearance of inulin, substituting and rearranging Equation 4-1:

$$\text{Phosphate reabsorbed} = \frac{U_{In} \cdot \dot{V}}{P_{In}} \cdot P_P - (U_P \cdot \dot{V}) \qquad (4\text{-}2)$$

A precise determination of the filtered quantity — often referred to as the "filtered load" — of any solute must correct for three factors: (a) the slightly higher concentration of the solute in plasma water than in whole plasma; (b) the effect of the Donnan equilibrium, which of course applies only to electrolytes; and (c) possible binding of the solute to plasma proteins, since the bound portion cannot be filtered. For many substances, these correction factors are small or nonexistent, and they frequently cancel out one another. Hence, the corrections have been ignored throughout this book. Nevertheless, it should be noted that most substances in the body are probably bound to plasma proteins; by and large, however, this is not true of the compounds considered in this text.

Problem 4-1 and its solution in the Answers section list raw data from an experiment that tested the characteristics of inorganic phosphate transport in the dog. A few of the derived values, converted from milligrams of phosphorus to millimoles of phosphate, are shown in Table 4-1, and they have been plotted in Figure 4-1.

Table 4-1
Renal handling of inorganic phosphate as a function of plasma phosphate concentration.

Plasma Phosphate Concentration (mM/L)	Filtered Load of Phosphate (mM/min)	Phosphate	
		Reabsorbed (mM/min)	Excreted (mM/min)
0.404	0.035	0.035	0
0.329	0.027	0.027	0
1.195	0.098	0.088	0.010
3.015	0.248	0.099	0.149
4.197	0.352	0.098	0.254
10.234	0.775	0.103	0.672

Transport Maximum (Tm)

Note that at low plasma concentrations all phosphate that is filtered is reabsorbed. Then the amount that is reabsorbed reaches a maximal value that does not vary even though more and more phosphate is filtered into Bowman's space. This constant value of reabsorbed phosphate, expressed as amount per minute, is known as the _transport maximum (Tm)_. Many other substances that are reabsorbed by the kidneys have a Tm. Examples include glucose and other sugars, sulfate, many amino acids, uric acid, and probably albumin.

Normally the plasma phosphate concentration in dogs and man is at a level where slightly more phosphate is filtered than the tubules can reabsorb. In other words, normally Tm for inorganic phosphate is exceeded, so that small amounts of phosphate are excreted.

Characteristics of Active Transport

Active transport may be defined as the net movement of a particle against an electrochemical potential gradient, at the

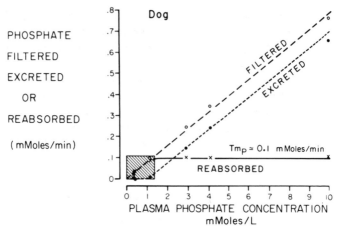

Figure 4-1
Renal filtration, reabsorption, and excretion of inorganic phosphate in dogs, plotted as a function of plasma phosphate concentration. The shaded area extends to the upper limit of normal plasma phosphate concentration; plasma phosphate exists mainly in two forms: $HPO_4^=$ and $H_2PO_4^-$ (see Fig. 9-5). Normally, small amounts of phosphate are excreted. Note that Tm_P refers to the maximal amount that the tubules can transport per unit time. Slightly modified from Pitts, R. F., and Alexander, R. S. *Amer. J. Physiol.* 142:648, 1944.

expense of metabolic energy. As shown in Equations 2-3 and 2-4, the net movement of an electrolyte may be down its chemical concentration gradient and still require energy if it has to move against a relatively higher electrical potential gradient; the converse, net movement down an electrical potential gradient but against a relatively greater chemical concentration gradient would also require energy and would therefore be called active.

Metabolic Inhibition. It follows from the above definition that if a system is deprived of metabolic energy, the net flux of an actively transported substance against its electrochemical potential gradient should be diminished or abolished. Such inhibition of transport is commonly seen if a system is cooled, or deprived of oxygen, or exposed to specific metabolic inhibitors such as dinitrophenol (DNP), which prevents the formation of high-energy phosphate bonds (see Figure 2-6).

Tm. The nonlinear relationship shown in Figure 4-1, between the plasma concentration of a given substance and its rate of transport, is another characteristic feature of many substances that are transported actively. The Tm phenomenon is apparently not due to exhaustion of the energy supply, but possibly to saturation of a hypothetical "carrier." For this reason, the term *saturation kinetics* is often used to describe the Tm phenomenon.

One possible scheme for visualizing active transport is depicted in Figure 4-2. Although the figure refers to a renal tubular cell, the diagram presumably applies to many other cells as well. A substance, S, is thought to combine with a "carrier," X, located within the cellular membrane. After traversing the membrane, the complex, S · X, dissociates, S moving passively through the cytoplasm and peritubular membrane into the peritubular fluid and blood. In this process, the carrier acquires a new form, Y, and it may be the reconversion of the carrier into its original form, which requires energy. Thus, in the net, the movement of S · X across the membrane is an energy-consuming process.

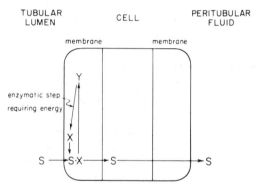

Figure 4-2
One hypothetical scheme for a carrier-mediated active transport system.

In some instances, S may first move passively through the luminal (apical, or mucosal) membrane and cytoplasm, and the energy-requiring step involving the complex may occur at the peritubular (basal, or serosal) membrane. While the system depicted in Figure 4-2 is compatible with experimental observations, it must be emphasized that the scheme is hypothetical. Despite extensive search, the carrier X has not been identified; it is not known whether or by what mechanism the complex S · X is formed, whether or how it is transported across the cell membrane, or by what mechanism the complex might be dissociated.

Competitive Inhibition. This is the process by which some substances can diminish the rate of transport of certain other substances, presumably by competing for attachment to the same carrier. For example, an intravenous infusion of fructose will diminish or abolish the tubular reabsorption of glucose. Similarly, many amino acids can compete against one another for what appears to be a common carrier system. The inhibitory effect of phlorizin on renal glucose reabsorption, referred to earlier, is probably a competitive phenomenon.

It must be emphasized that substances that are actively transported do not necessarily manifest all these characteristics. For example, in Chapter 7 we present the experimental evidence that Na^+ can be transported against an electrochemical potential gradient, not only by renal tubular cells but also by most other cells. Although this process requires energy (see Fig. 2-6), a Tm for Na^+ has not been demonstrated. Furthermore, the carrier concept and saturation kinetics are not limited to active transport, for in some instances passive transport processes may also be carrier-mediated.

Glucose Titration Curve

The glucose titration curve is constructed by determining the amount of glucose that is reabsorbed at increasing plasma glucose concentrations. If the GFR stays constant, increasing the plasma concentration of glucose will lead to a progressive rise in the filtered load of glucose (GFR $\cdot$ P_G), i.e., in the amount of glucose presented to the proximal tubules for reabsorption. In this way, the system is titrated to determine the plasma concentration at which the "carrier" for glucose becomes saturated and glucose is spilled in the urine.

A typical glucose titration curve in man is presented in Figure 4-3. It is apparent that the curve has the form that is characteristic of a Tm-limited active transport system; in fact, it was the first renal Tm-limited system to be described. At first, virtually all the filtered glucose is reabsorbed and 0.1% or less of that which was filtered is excreted. This is the case at normal plasma glucose concentrations, as denoted by the shaded rectangle. Then, as the maximal capacity of the tubules for reabsorbing glucose is reached, much more glucose is excreted in the urine. (In the experiment shown in Fig. 4-3, the amount filtered, and hence that which was excreted, fell off slightly at higher plasma concentrations because the GFR decreased slightly.)

Splay

Note that Tm for glucose is approached somewhat gradually, along a curve, rather than abruptly with a sharp deflection. The curve is known as the *splay*, and it probably has at least two explanations. The first involves the kinetics of the chemical

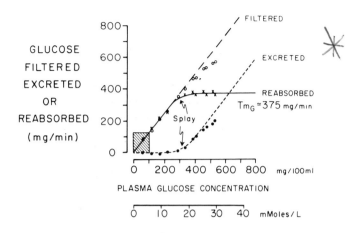

GLUCOSE
FILTERED
EXCRETED
OR
REABSORBED
(mg/min)

FILTERED

EXCRETED

REABSORBED
$Tm_G \approx 375$ mg/min

Splay

PLASMA GLUCOSE CONCENTRATION

C_{in} decreased slowly from 122 to 100 ml/min

Figure 4-3
Renal handling of glucose as a function of increasing plasma glucose concentrations. The curve for reabsorption is known as the glucose titration curve because it determines the plasma concentration at which the "carrier" for glucose becomes saturated. Note that Tm_G refers to the maximal amount of glucose that can be transported per unit time. Normal plasma glucose concentrations (70 to 100 mg/100 ml) fall within the shaded square; thus, normally virtually all the filtered glucose is re-absorbed. The significance of the splay is explained in the text. In the clinical laboratory, plasma glucose concentrations are ordinarily expressed as milligrams per 100 ml of plasma; corresponding concentrations, in millimoles per liter, are given on the second abscissa. Data from Smith, H. W. *Principles of Renal Physiology.* Oxford University Press, New York, 1956.

reaction between glucose and the postulated carrier. To the extent that the carrier has a finite affinity for glucose, a "supersaturating" concentration of glucose in the tubular fluid will be needed to saturate the carrier. Hence, glucose will be spilled in the urine before Tm is reached, and some splay will result.

The second explanation involves the concept of morphological glomerulotubular balance (G-T balance). It has been shown that there is considerable variation in the anatomical dimensions of glomeruli and renal tubules. In any one person, for example, there may be an 8-fold difference in the glomerular surface area available for filtration, and a twofold to threefold variation in the volume of the proximal tubule. Unless the glucose reabsorptive capacity of each proximal tubule is tailored precisely to the glucose filtering capacity of its own glomerulus, some nephrons will excrete glucose before Tm_G for most nephrons is reached, and other nephrons will continue to reabsorb glucose after Tm_G has been exceeded in most nephrons. Thus, the degree of splay in the glucose titration curve partly reflects the extent of anatomical G-T balance. The fact that this splay is small means that the balance is remarkably precise, so that despite the great variation in anatomical dimensions the balance between filtering and reabsorptive capacity in the majority of individual nephrons is similar to this balance for the kidney as a whole.

The concept of G-T balance is not limited to glucose, but may be applied to all substances that are filtered and reabsorbed. Furthermore, the term *glomerulotubular* balance is used in two contexts: (a) when comparing the amount of a substance filtered with the *maximal* capacity of the tubular system to reabsorb that substance, as in the case of glucose and (b) when comparing the amount of a substance filtered with the *fraction* of the filtered load that the tubules reabsorb. The latter meaning has special significance for Na^+ balance and it is discussed in detail in Chapter 7.

Passive Reabsorption: Urea

The influence of acute changes in the rate of urine flow on the urinary excretion of urea is shown in Figure 4-4a. The rate of excretion increases markedly with increments in urine flow up to about 2 ml per minute, and thereafter it increases at a lesser rate. The increased excretion could be due to an increase in the amount of urea filtered (GFR $\cdot$ P_U) or to decreased reabsorption of urea, or to a combination of the two. Since the plasma concentration of urea and the GFR stayed relatively constant in the experiment depicted in Figure 4-4, the filtered load of urea did not change; hence the increased excretion with rising urine flows must have been due to decreased tubular reabsorption, as depicted in Figure 4-4b.

 The relationship between the rate of urine flow and the reabsorptive rate for urea is characteristic of a substance that undergoes passive tubular reabsorption. The increase in urine flow shown in Figure 4-4 was due to decreased reabsorption of water from the distal tubules and collecting ducts; that is, there was increased flow of tubular fluid, mainly water, in the distal convolutions and collecting ducts. Consequently, the concentration of urea in these tubular structures, and hence the difference in urea concentration between tubular and interstitial fluid, declined. Since passive transport of a nonelectrolyte depends

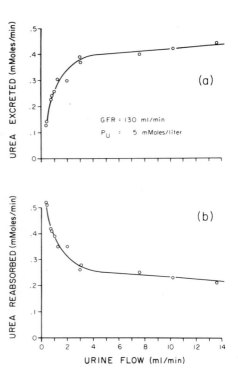

Figure 4-4
(a) An experiment in man showing the influence of the rate of urine flow on urea excretion. The points represent values in a single individual in whom urine flow was decreased by withdrawing drinking water, and subsequently increased by ingesting large amounts of water. Since the filtered load of urea $(GFR \cdot P_U)$ did not change with increasing urine flow, the increased excretion must have been due to decreased reabsorption (Eq. 4-1); this fact is shown in (b). Data adapted from Austin, J. H., Stillman, E., and Van Slyke, D. D. *J. Biol. Chem.* 46:91, 1921.

largely on its chemical concentration gradient, the reabsorption of urea decreased. The decline in the reabsorptive rate is much steeper at low than at high urine flows because the concentration gradient, i.e., the driving force for passive reabsorption, decreases more per linear unit rise in urine flow at low flow rates that it does at high flow rates.

Having emphasized the importance of urea as a solute that is passively reabsorbed, it must now be admitted that a small portion of that which is filtered may be actively reabsorbed by the mammalian nephron. Under most physiological conditions, however, the majority probably is reabsorbed passively. To compound the confusion, urea is actively secreted by some amphibians and, as discussed below, it is passively secreted into the loops of Henle of mammals.

Bidirectional Transport

Equation 4-1 can give a measure only of *net* reabsorption. When we describe the renal handling of a substance as involving filtration and reabsorption, we mean filtration followed by net flux from tubular lumen to blood. The statement does not exclude the possibility that the substance is simultaneously secreted, i.e., moved from blood into tubular fluid. In fact, for many or most substances, net tubular reabsorption or net secretion is the algebraic sum of fluxes in both directions; and the mode of transport in any one direction may be passive or active, or a combination of the two. For example, Na^+ undergoes net reabsorption, but it moves across the tubular wall in two directions, being actively reabsorbed and passively secreted.

Some substances undergo net transport in one direction in one part of the nephron, and net movement in the opposite direction in another part. Thus, K^+ (Chap. 11) is usually reabsorbed in the proximal tubules and loops of Henle, secreted in the distal tubules, and reabsorbed in the collecting ducts. For the entire kidney, there may be net reabsorption or net secretion of K^+, depending on the conditions. Certain weak acids and bases, including many drugs such as the antimalarials and salicylate (a metabolic product of aspirin), undergo active secretion in the proximal tubule and passive reabsorption predominantly in the distal tubule.

There are also a number of compounds that undergo either net reabsorption or net secretion through carrier-mediated processes in the same tubular segment. For example, uric acid is thought to be both reabsorbed and secreted in this manner, in the proximal tubule, the net movement in one direction or the other depending on a variety of experimental conditions.

In the preceding section, we stressed the reabsorption of urea from the distal tubules and collecting ducts. Actually the renal handling of *urea* is much more complicated. The scheme shown in Figure 4-5 is based on micropuncture studies, mainly in rats, at normal rates of urine flow. The numbers within the lumen denote the percentage of the filtered load of urea that flows at the various sites. About 50% of the filtered urea is reabsorbed in the proximal tubules. Yet, 100% or more of the filtered amount of urea is found at the beginning of the distal tubules; therefore, urea must diffuse into the intermediate segments, i.e., the loops of Henle and possibly the late proximal tubules. At normal rates of urine flow, urea is then again reabsorbed in the distal convolutions and collecting ducts, so that about 40% of the filtered load of urea is excreted. Thus, urea also exhibits bidirectional transport. It undergoes net reabsorption from the proximal tubules, distal tubules, and collecting ducts, and it undergoes net secretion into the loops of Henle and possibly into the pars recta of the proximal tubules. The possible advantage of

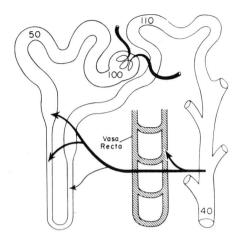

Figure 4-5
Renal handling of urea at normal rates of urine flow. The numbers within
the lumen denote the percentage of the filtered amount of urea that flows
at the various sites. The urea that is reabsorbed from the collecting ducts
flows partly into the vasa recta, and partly into the tubular segments that
lie between the late proximal and early distal tubules. This process is called
"medullary recycling of urea." Data adapted from Lassiter, W. E.,
Gottschalk, C. W., and Mylle, M. *Amer. J. Physiol.* 200:1139, 1961.

this seemingly complicated handling of urea, for the process of
urinary concentration, is considered in Chapter 8.

Summary

The term *tubular reabsorption* refers to the direction of tubular
transport, from tubular lumen, through peritubular interstitium,
into blood. This definition applies to all modes of transport in the
reabsorptive direction. Many of the compounds that undergo net
tubular reabsorption are essential to homeostasis, e.g., Na^+,
HCO_3^-, H_2O, glucose, and amino acids.

When we speak of a compound as being handled by filtration
and reabsorption, we usually mean filtration followed by *net*
reabsorption; such net transport can be deduced from Equation
4-1 as the difference between the amount filtered and that which
is excreted in the urine.

Many substances, such as Na^+, inorganic phosphate, and
glucose are actively reabsorbed, i.e., against an electrochemical
potential gradient at the expense of metabolic energy. Many such
compounds exhibit the characteristic features of active transport:
metabolic inhibition, transport maximum (Tm), and competitive

inhibition. Na^+, however, exhibits no Tm even though it is actively reabsorbed. The degree of splay in a curve showing Tm (e.g., the glucose titration curve) is probably a function of two phenomena: (a) affinity of the "carrier" for the transported substance; and (b) anatomical glomerulotubular (G-T) balance.

The rate of tubular reabsorption of urea, which in mammals is mainly by passive diffusion, varies as a function of the rate of urine flow. Like many other compounds, urea exhibits bidirectional transport; it undergoes net reabsorption in the proximal tubules, distal tubules, and collecting ducts, and net secretion into the loops of Henle and possibly the pars recta.

Problem 4-1. Renal handling of inorganic phosphate in dogs. Utilizing the data given, complete the blank columns.

| Urine Flow (ml/min) | Phosphate Phosphorus[a] | | | Creatinine | | | Phosphate Phosphorus[a] | | | Ratio: Phosphate Clearance/ Creatinine Clearance |
	Plasma (mg/100 ml)	Urine (mg/100 ml)	Clearance (ml/min)	Plasma (mg/100 ml)	Urine (mg/100 ml)	Clearance (ml/min)	Filtered (mg/min)	Excreted (mg/min)	Reabsorbed (mg/min)	
6.8	1.25	0.07		33.9	427					
6.8	1.16	0.08		32.0	392					
7.0	1.02	0.08		31.3	367					
9.2	2.75	0.46		31.2	283					
9.7	3.70	2.95		32.5	274					
8.7	4.64	9.10		33.3	321					
6.7	9.34	69.0		34.5	423					
7.6	11.6	83.6		34.3	375					
8.2	13.0	95.7		34.5	352					
9.2	23.9	171		36.9	313					
10.0	27.9	184		37.7	294					
10.0	31.7	208		38.7	293					

[a]The values were measured as phosphate phosphorus; they have been converted from milligrams to millimoles of inorganic phosphate in Table 4-1 and Figure 4-1.

Slightly modified from Pitts, R. F., and Alexander, R. S. *Amer. J. Physiol.* 142:648, 1944. Used with permission of the American Physiological Society.

Problem 4-2. Handling of urea by the kidneys of adult man at varying rates of urine flow. Utilizing the data given, complete the blank columns.

| V̇ (ml/min) | Urine Concentration | | Plasma Concentration | | GFR (ml/min) | Urea | | | Urea | |
	Inulin (mg/ml)	Urea (mM/L)	Inulin (mg/ml)	Urea (mM/L)		Filtered (mM/min)	Excreted (mM/min)	Reabsorbed (mM/min)	Excreted	Reabsorbed (% of filtered load)
0.4	144	300	0.5	5						
0.8	75	263	0.5	5						
1.0	60	240	0.5	5						
3.1	20	119	0.5	5						
10.2	5.8	37	0.5	5						

Selected References

General

Forster, R. P. Renal transport mechanisms. *Fed. Proc.* 26:1008, 1967.

Lotspeich, W. D. *Metabolic Aspects of Renal Function.* Thomas, Springfield, Ill., 1959.

Mudge, G. H., Berndt, W. O., and Valtin, H. Tubular Transport of Urea, Glucose, Phosphate, Uric Acid, Sulfate, and Thiosulfate. In J. Orloff and R. W. Berliner (Eds.), *Handbook of Physiology.* Section 8: Renal Physiology. American Physiological Society, Washington, D.C., 1973.

Pitts, R. F. *Physiology of the Kidney and Body Fluids,* 2d ed. Year Book, Chicago, 1968. Chap. 6.

Smith, H. W. *The Kidney: Structure and Function in Health and Disease.* Oxford University Press, New York, 1951.

Stein, W. D. *The Movement of Molecules Across Cell Membranes.* Academic, New York, 1967.

Wearn, J. T., and Richards, A. N. Observations on the composition of glomerular urine with particular reference to the problem of reabsorption in the renal tubules. *Amer. J. Physiol.* 71:209, 1924.

Glucose

Bradley, S. E., Laragh, J. H., Wheeler, H. O., MacDowell, M., and Oliver, J. Correlation of structure and function in the handling of glucose by nephrons of the canine kidney. *J. Clin. Invest.* 40:1113, 1961.

Davison, J. M., and Cheyne, G. A. Renal reabsorption of glucose. *Lancet* 1:787, 1972.

Frohnert, P. P., Höhmann, B., Zwiebel, R., and Baumann, K. Free flow micropuncture studies of glucose transport in the rat nephron. *Pflügers Eur. J. Physiol.* 315:66, 1970.

Lotspeich, W. D. *Phlorizin and the Cellular Transport of Glucose.* The Harvey Lectures, Series LVI, 1960–61. Academic, New York, 1961.

Oliver, J., and MacDowell, M. The structural and functional aspects of the handling of glucose by the nephrons and the kidney and their correlation by means of structural-functional equivalents. *J. Clin. Invest.* 40:1093, 1961.

Rohde, R., and Deetjen, P. Die Glucoseresorption in der Rattenniere. Mikropunktionsanalysen der tubulären Glucosekonzentration bei freiem Fluss. *Pflügers Arch. Ges. Physiol.* 302:219, 1968.

Shannon, J. A., and Fisher, S. The renal tubular reabsorption of glucose in the normal dog. *Amer. J. Physiol.* 122:765, 1938.

Silverman, M., Aganon, M. A., and Chinard, F. P. Specificity of monosaccharide transport in dog kidney. *Amer. J. Physiol.* 218:743, 1970.

Smith, H., Goldring, W., Chasis, H., Ranges, H. A., and Bradley, S. E. The application of saturation methods to the study of glomerular and tubular function in the human kidney. *J. Mount Sinai Hosp.* (N.Y.) 10:59, 1943.

van Liew, J. B., Deetjen, P., and Boylan, J. W. Glucose reabsorption in the rat kidney: Dependence on glomerular filtration. *Pflügers Arch. Ges. Physiol.* 295:232, 1967.

Urea and
Uric Acid

Clapp, J. Renal tubular reabsorption of urea in normal and protein-depleted rats. *Amer. J. Physiol.* 210:1304, 1966.

Forster, R. Active cellular transport of urea by frog renal tubules. *Amer. J. Physiol.* 179:372, 1954.

Goldberg, M., Wojtczak, A. M., and Ramirez, M. A. Uphill transport of urea in the dog kidney: Effects of certain inhibitors. *J. Clin. Invest.* 46:388, 1967.

Lassiter, W. E., Gottschalk, C. W., and Mylle, M. Micropuncture study of net transtubular movement of water and urea in nondiuretic mammalian kidney. *Amer. J. Physiol.* 200:1139, 1961.

Lassiter, W. E., Mylle, M., and Gottschalk, C. W. Net transtubular movement of water and urea in saline diuresis. *Amer. J. Physiol.* 206:669, 1964.

Lassiter, W. E., Mylle, M., and Gottschalk, C. W. Micropuncture study of urea transport in rat renal medulla. *Amer. J. Physiol.* 210:965, 1966.

May, D. G., and Weiner, I. M. The renal mechanisms for the excretion of m-hydroxybenzoic acids in *Cebus* monkeys: Relationship to urate transport. *J. Pharmacol. Exp. Ther.* 176:407, 1971.

Mudge, G. H., Berndt, W. O., and Valtin, H. Tubular Transport of Urea, Glucose, Phosphate, Uric Acid, Sulfate, and Thiosulfate. In J. Orloff and R. W. Berliner (Eds.), *Handbook of Physiology.* Section 8: Renal Physiology. American Physiological Society, Washington, D.C., 1973.

Schmidt-Nielsen, B. Urea excretion in mammals. *Physiol. Rev.* 38:139, 1958.

Schmidt-Nielsen, B. (Ed.). *Urea and the Kidney.* Excerpta Medica Foundation, Amsterdam, 1970.

Shannon, J. A. Urea excretion in the normal dog during forced diuresis. *Amer. J. Physiol.* 122:782, 1938.

Ullrich, K. J., Rumrich, G., and Baldamus, C. A. Mode of Urea Transport Across the Mammalian Nephron. In B. Schmidt-Nielsen (Ed.), *Urea and the Kidney.* Excerpta Medica Foundation, Amsterdam, 1970.

Phosphate

Hellman, D., Baird, H. R., and Bartter, F. C. Relationship of maximal tubular phosphate reabsorption to filtration rate in the dog. *Amer. J. Physiol.* 207:89, 1964.

Mudge, G. H., Berndt, W. O., and Valtin, H. Tubular Transport of Urea, Glucose, Phosphate, Uric Acid, Sulfate and Thiosulfate. In J. Orloff and R. W. Berliner (Eds.), *Handbook of Physiology.* Section 8: Renal Physiology. American Physiological Society, Washington, D.C., 1973.

Pitts, R. F., and Alexander, R. S. The renal reabsorptive mechanism for inorganic phosphate in normal and acidotic dogs. *Amer. J. Physiol.* 142:648, 1944.

Strickler, J. C., Thompson, D. D., Klose, R. M., and Giebisch, G. Micropuncture study of inorganic phosphate excretion in the rat. *J. Clin. Invest.* 43:1596, 1964.

Sulfate

Lotspeich, W. D. Renal tubular reabsorption of inorganic sulfate in the normal dog. *Amer. J. Physiol.* 151:311, 1947.

Mudge, G. H., Berndt, W. O., and Valtin, H. Tubular Transport of Urea, Glucose, Phosphate, Uric Acid, Sulfate and Thiosulfate. In J. Orloff and R. W. Berliner (Eds.), *Handbook of Physiology.* Section 8: Renal Physiology. American Physiological Society, Washington, D.C., 1973.

Amino Acids and Proteins

Beyer, K. H., Wright, L. D., Skeggs, H. R., Russo, H. F., and Shaner, G. A. Renal clearance of essential amino acids: Their competition for reabsorption by the renal tubules. *Amer. J. Physiol.* 151:202, 1947.

Brown, J. L., Samiy, A. H., and Pitts, R. F. Localization of amino-nitrogen reabsorption in the nephron of the dog. *Amer. J. Physiol.* 200:370, 1961.

Cortney, M. A., Sawin, L. L., and Weiss, D. D. Renal tubular protein absorption in the rat. *J. Clin. Invest.* 49:1, 1970.

Cusworth, D. C., and Dent, C. E. Renal clearances of amino acids in normal adults and in patients with aminoaciduria. *Biochem. J.* 74:550, 1960.

Kamin, H., and Handler, P. Effect of infusion of single amino acids upon excretion of other amino acids. *Amer. J. Physiol.* 164:654, 1951.

Leber, P. D., and Marsh, D. J. Micropuncture study of concentration and fate of albumin in rat nephron. *Amer. J. Physiol.* 219:358, 1970.

Maunsbach, A. B. Absorption of I^{125}-labeled homologous albumin by rat kidney proximal tubule cells: A study of microperfused single proximal tubules by electron microscopic autoradiography and histochemistry. *J. Ultrastruct. Res.* 15:197, 1966.

Oken, D. E., Cotes, S. C., and Mende, C. W. Micropuncture study of tubular transport of albumin in rats with aminonucleoside nephrosis. *Kidney Int.* 1:3, 1972.

Robson, E. B., and Rose, G. A. The effect of intravenous lysine on the renal clearances of cystine, arginine and ornithine in normal subjects, in patients with cystinuria and Fanconi syndrome and in their relatives. *Clin. Sci.* 16:75, 1957.

Rosenberg, L. E., Downing, S. J., and Segal, S. Competitive inhibition of dibasic amino acid transport in rat kidney. *J. Biol. Chem.* 237:2265, 1962.

Scriver, C. R. Renal tubular transport of proline, hydroxyproline, and glycine: III. Genetic basis for more than one mode of transport in human kidney. *J. Clin. Invest.* 47:823, 1968.

Segal, S., and Thiere, S. O. The Renal Handling of Amino Acids. In J. Orloff and R. W. Berliner (Eds.), *Handbook of Physiology.* Section 8: Renal Physiology. American Physiological Society, Washington, D.C., 1973.

Strickler, J. C., and Frimpter, G. W. Renal excretion of cystathionine in dogs. *Amer. J. Physiol.* 217:1199, 1969.

Webber, W. A., Brown, J. L., and Pitts, R. F. Interactions of amino acids in renal tubular transport. *Amer. J. Physiol.* 200:380, 1961.

Wilson, O. H., and Scriver, C. R. Specificity of transport of neutral and basic amino acids in rat kidney. *Amer. J. Physiol.* 213:185, 1967.

5 : Tubular Secretion

The term *secretion* refers to the *direction* of movement, from peritubular blood, or interstitium, or tubular cell into the tubular lumen, regardless of whether the transport is passive or active. The term excludes entry of substances into the tubular lumen via glomerular filtration.

Many of the substances that are secreted by renal tubules are either weak acids or weak bases, and many fall into one or more of the following categories. (1) They are foreign to the body. Drugs, such as penicillin and salicylate (a breakdown product of aspirin), are examples; H^+ and NH_3 are notable exceptions. (2) They are not metabolized, but are excreted unchanged in the urine, e.g., para-aminohippuric acid (PAH). (3) They are metabolized slowly, incompletely, and with difficulty, e.g., thiamine (vitamin B_1). Thus, tubular secretion may be viewed as a supplement to glomerular filtration, to help in the elimination of compounds that cannot be disposed of by metabolism alone.

The fact that secreted substances are mainly compounds that are foreign to the body has often raised the question whether the tubular secretory mechanism normally plays any essential physiological role. Julius Cohen and his associates have suggested that one such role may be the acquisition, by renal cells, of essential metabolic substrates. For example, α-ketoglutarate is selectively taken up by the kidneys and the liver, and it is actively transported across the basilar membrane, from the blood into renal and hepatic cells. It may be a mere concomitant resulting from structural similarity that foreign organic compounds such as PAH can utilize the same carrier mechanism and thus be efficiently excreted by the kidney.

Qualitative Evidence for Secretion

The possibility that some substances might be secreted was vehemently rejected for a long time. As mentioned in Chapter 1, Cushny regarded the process of tubular secretion to be so vitalistic as to be inconceivable. (In an introductory letter to the monograph, in which Cushny presented his view, he stated: "If it [the monograph] serves as an advanced post from which others may issue against the remaining ramparts of vitalism, its purpose will be served." It is an ironic twist that Cushny entitled the monograph, *The Secretion of the Urine*; the definition of secretion that is given above was introduced after the appearance of Cushny's book.)

The first convincing evidence for tubular secretion appeared in 1923, when E. K. Marshall, Jr., and J. L. Vickers showed that as much as 70% of an injected dye, phenolsulfonphthalein (PSP), could appear in the urine in a single circulation through the kidneys. Since about 75% of PSP is bound to plasma proteins, only 25% was available for filtration; hence about 45% of the injected PSP must have reached the urine by secretion. Those who objected to the concept of tubular secretion, however, pointed out that PSP is a foreign substance and that Marshall's demonstration therefore might have little physiological meaning. Five years later, Marshall and A. L. Grafflin showed that endogenous compounds such as creatine and creatinine, were excreted in the urine of the goosefish, *Lophius,* which has virtually no glomeruli. Nevertheless, this report was purportedly met by some obstinate skeptics with the comment that ". . . at last Marshall has found an animal that fits in with his theory."

Tubular secretion was subsequently demonstrated in numerous animals and preparations. For example, it was shown by direct visualization that PSP could be concentrated several thousandfold within the lumina of separated tubules without glomeruli, and that this accumulation could be prevented by the metabolic poison, dinitrophenol (DNP), or by depriving the preparation of oxygen. Thus, the secretion of at least some substances must be an active transport process. The reality of tubular secretion became fully accepted with the development of the inulin clearance as a means of quantifying the rate of glomerular filtration. With this tool, as is shown in Equation 5-1, it could be clearly shown in vivo, that the rate of urinary excretion of many substances far exceeded the rate at which they are filtered.

Quantifying Secretion

The calculation is based on the following equation:

Quantity excreted = quantity filtered + quantity secreted   (5-1)

For PAH:

$$\text{Quantity excreted} = U_{PAH} \cdot \dot{V}$$

$$\text{Quantity filtered} = P_{PAH} \cdot C_{In}$$

where U_{PAH} = the concentration of PAH in the urine (mg/ml)

$\dot{V}$ = the rate of urine flow (ml/min)

P_{PAH} = the concentration of PAH in the plasma (mg/ml). (Strictly speaking, this concentration should be corrected for several factors, including the binding of PAH to plasma proteins; but, as stated in conjunction with Equation 4-2, these corrections will be ignored.)

C_{In} = the clearance of inulin, i.e., GFR (ml/min).

Substituting, and rearranging Equation 5-1:

$$\text{Quantity of PAH secreted} = (U_{PAH} \cdot \dot{V}) - \left(P_{PAH} \cdot \frac{U_{In} \cdot \dot{V}}{P_{In}} \right) \qquad (5\text{-}2)$$

PAH is actively secreted by the proximal tubules, from the peritubular blood into the tubular lumen. We might therefore anticipate a secretory transport maximum, Tm, for PAH. The existence of this maximum is shown in Figure 5-1, which depicts the handling of PAH by the kidneys of a normal adult man as the plasma concentration of PAH is raised progressively by intravenous infusion. Note that, at plasma concentrations above 20 mg/100 ml, PAH secretion becomes constant because Tm_{PAH} has been reached. In normal man, the maximal amount of PAH that can be transported by all proximal tubular cells combined is about 80 mg per minute.

Measurement of Renal Plasma Flow

In Chapter 3 we stressed that only about one-fifth of the plasma that enters the glomerular capillaries can be filtered into Bowman's space. Inulin can get into the tubular system only by filtration, i.e., as a solute dissolved in plasma. It follows, therefore, that only about one-fifth of the inulin can be removed

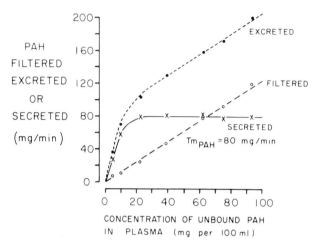

Figure 5-1
Rates of filtration, excretion, and secretion of para-aminohippuric acid (PAH) in man, at increasing plasma concentrations of PAH. The plasma concentrations refer to that portion of the PAH that is not bound to plasma proteins and that is therefore freely filterable. Slightly modified from Pitts, R. F. *Physiology of the Kidney and Body Fluids,* 2d ed. Year Book, Chicago, 1968.

from the plasma as blood courses through the kidneys at any one time. However, a substance like PAH, which besides being filtered also undergoes active tubular secretion, can be almost "completely" removed. This has been proved by simultaneously sampling arterial and renal venous blood; as the blood enters the kidney, it has a finite concentration of PAH, and as the blood leaves the kidney, the concentration is virtually zero. "Complete" removal is possible because the substance does not need to be dissolved in plasma in order to be secreted into the tubular lumen; it can be transported by the "carrier" without plasma.

Obviously, "complete" removal in a single circuit of the blood through the kidneys is possible only if the secretory Tm for PAH has not been reached. Consequently, the procedure for *estimating* renal plasma flow with PAH is as follows:

1. Infuse PAH intravenously at a rate that will result in a steady, low plasma concentration that will not saturate the secretory transport mechanism, i.e., which will maintain the rate of secretion well below Tm.
2. Measure the concentration of PAH in the urine; U_{PAH} = 25.5 mg/ml.
3. Measure the rate of urine flow; $\dot{V}$ = 1.1 ml/min.
4. Calculate the rate of urinary excretion of PAH; $U_{PAH} \cdot \dot{V}$ = 28 mg/min.

5. Measure the concentration of PAH in arterial plasma; P_{PAH} = 0.05 mg/ml.

6. If each milliliter of plasma flowing through the glomeruli and peritubular vessels contributed 0.05 mg of PAH to the urine (which must be so if the renal venous concentration of PAH is zero), how many milliliters of plasma must have passed through the kidneys in order to have excreted 28 mg of PAH?

$$28 \text{ mg} \div \frac{0.05 \text{ mg}}{\text{ml}} = \frac{28 \text{ mg}}{1} \cdot \frac{\text{ml}}{0.05 \text{ mg}} = 560 \text{ ml}$$

Since 28 mg was excreted in one minute, 560 ml of plasma must have passed through the kidneys during this one minute. Note that we have calculated the clearance of PAH, $U_{PAH} \cdot \dot{V}/P_{PAH}$.

Concept of Effective Renal Plasma Flow (ERPF)

In the above description, the word *complete* has been in quotation marks because actually the concentration of PAH in renal venous blood is not zero but rather about one-tenth of its concentration in renal arterial blood. This is probably so because some blood flows through renal tissue that does not remove PAH, e.g., the renal capsule, the renal pelvis, the perirenal fat, and possibly the outer medulla and papilla. Since the procedure described above measures the flow that traverses tissue that *effectively* removes PAH from the plasma, the rate of flow thus determined is called the *effective renal plasma flow* (ERPF). Hence, at low plasma concentration of PAH, the clearance of PAH is a measure of ERPF.

$$C_{PAH} = \frac{U_{PAH} \cdot \dot{V}}{P_{PAH}} = \text{ERPF (ml/min)} \qquad (5\text{-}3)$$

Extraction of PAH: Exact Renal Plasma Flow (RPF)

By simultaneously measuring the concentration of PAH in renal arterial and renal venous plasma, one can determine exactly how much PAH was extracted from each milliliter of plasma flowing through the kidneys. In this way one can precisely measure the renal plasma flow (RPF), as opposed to the ERPF. In fact, whenever an exact determination of RPF is needed, the extraction of PAH is measured. This is necessary not only because under control conditions only 85 to 90% is extracted, but also because the rate of extraction can vary by 20% or more during various physiological and experimental conditions. This fact, and sample calculations of RPF using the extraction of PAH, are given in Problem 5-1 and in the corresponding Answer.

Moreover, one can measure RPF precisely by determining the extraction of any one of a number of substances. This point can be illustrated for urea. If the urinary concentration of urea is 12 mg per milliliter, and the urine flow is 1.1 ml per minute, the urinary excretion of urea is 13.2 mg per minute. If, while this excretion rate was measured, the concentration of urea in renal arterial plasma was 0.26 mg per milliliter, and that in renal venous plasma was 0.24 mg per milliliter, each milliliter of plasma traversing the kidneys must have contributed 0.02 mg to the 13.2 mg that was excreted. Hence the RPF must have been

$$\frac{13.2 \text{ mg}}{\text{min}} \div \frac{0.02 \text{ mg}}{\text{ml}} = \frac{13.2 \text{ mg}}{\text{min}} \cdot \frac{\text{ml}}{0.02 \text{ mg}} = 660 \text{ ml/min} = RPF$$

It will be apparent that this method of measuring RPF is an application of the Fick principle (see Eq. 6-1). The urinary excretion of urea is in a sense the renal consumption of urea and thus analogous to the $\dot{V}_{O_2}$ of Equation 6-1; and the concentration of 0.02 mg per milliliter is the difference between the renal arterial and renal venous concentrations of urea and is thus analogous to the a-v oxygen difference of Equation 6-1. Thus, the formula for measuring RPF by substance X (be it PAH, or urea, or some other substance) is:

$$RPF = \frac{U_X \cdot \dot{V}}{Pa_X - Pv_X} \tag{5-4}$$

where Pa_X = the concentration of substance X in renal arterial plasma

Pv_X = the concentration of X in renal venous plasma.

Extraction Ratio (E). This is the fraction of a given substance that is removed from the plasma in a single passage through the kidneys. It is calculated by the following equation:

$$E = \frac{Pa_X - Pv_X}{Pa_X} \tag{5-5}$$

The ratio can be calculated for any substance. For PAH at low plasma concentrations, Pv_{PAH} approaches zero, and E is about 0.85 to 0.90; for glucose, which is normally almost completely reabsorbed, E will be virtually 0.

From Equation 5-5, $E \cdot Pa_X = Pa_X - Pv_X$; substituting in Equation 5-4:

$$RPF = \frac{U_X \cdot \dot{V}}{Pa_X \cdot E} \qquad (5\text{-}6)$$

Catheterization of the renal artery and vein is now a fairly routine, safe procedure that is frequently done, even in unanesthetized human patients. The procedure is usually carried out for diagnostic purposes other than the determination of RPF, however. In most studies on humans, renal plasma flow is either measured by some method other than the Fick principle (see Chap. 6) or it is approximated as ERPF (Eq. 5-3). But in experimental work on animals, the Fick principle and Equation 5-6 are commonly employed. For a substance such as PAH, which is not metabolized by any organ, and not excreted by any organ other than the kidneys, a sample from any peripheral vessel can be used to determine Pa_X.

Calculation of Renal Blood Flow (RBF)

If the hematocrit (Hct) — i.e., the fraction of whole blood that is cells — is 0.45 or 45%, the fraction of whole blood that is plasma is 0.55. Hence,

$$\frac{RPF}{0.55} = \frac{RBF}{1.00} \text{ , and}$$

$$RBF = \frac{RPF}{0.55} = \frac{RPF}{1.00 - Hct} \qquad (5\text{-}7)$$

Substituting 660 ml per minute for RPF,

$$RBF = \frac{660}{1.00 - 0.45} = \frac{660}{0.55} = 1,200 \text{ ml/min}$$

Filtration Fraction (FF)

The filtration fraction, alluded to in Chapter 3, is that fraction of the plasma flowing through the kidneys that is filtered into

Bowman's space. It is calculated by the following formula:

$$FF = \frac{GFR}{RPF}$$

Substituting 132 ml per minute for GFR (see Fig. 3-3) and 660 ml per minute for RPF (above)

$$FF = \frac{132}{660} = 0.20$$

This is simply restating that normally about one-fifth, or 20%, of the plasma entering the glomerular capillaries is filtered.

Summary

Tubular secretion refers to the tranport of substances into the tubular lumen by means other than glomerular filtration. Secretion defines the direction of transport, not the mode. When we speak of a substance as being filtered and secreted, we usually mean *net* secretion; this net transport can be quantified by means of Equation 5-1.

At low plasma concentrations — i.e., below Tm_{PAH} — 85 to 90% of the PAH is removed from the plasma in a single circuit through the kidneys. Hence, at low plasma concentrations of PAH, the clearance of PAH, C_{PAH}, yields a fairly close approximation of the renal plasma flow; this approximation is known as the effective renal plasma flow (ERPF). The exact renal plasma flow (RPF) can be determined through application of the Fick principle, and this is often done by measuring the renal extraction of PAH.

The rate of renal blood flow (RBF) can be calculated by means of a simple proportionality if the fraction of whole blood that is made up of cells (the hematocrit) is known.

The filtration fraction (FF) is normally about 0.20; that is, normally about 20% of the plasma that traverses the kidneys is filtered into Bowman's space.

Problem 5-1. Determination of renal plasma flow (RPF), renal blood flow (RBF), and filtration fraction (FF), using PAH and inulin in dogs. The extraction ratio of PAH (E_{PAH}) changes during the postnatal period, during which these data were obtained. Utilizing the data given, fill in the blank columns.

Age (days)	Urine Flow (μl per min per g of kidney)[c]	U_{PAH} (mg/100 ml)	Pa_{PAH}[a] (mg/100 ml)	Pv_{PAH}[a] (mg/100 ml)	E_{PAH}	RPF (μl per min per g of kidney)[c]	RBF[b] (μl per min per g of kidney)[c]	C_{In} (μl per min per g of kidney)[c]	FF
2	3.8	104	2.60	2.16				130	
21	2.7	283	1.70	1.08				270	
40	5.2	664	3.00	1.23				630	
60	3.2	672	1.20	0.34				790	
74	2.3	3,516	3.10	0.52				1,200	

[a] Pa_{PAH} and Pv_{PAH} = concentration of PAH in arterial and renal venous plasma, respectively.

[b] Assume that the hematocrit = 0.45.

[c] Values have been expressed per gram of kidney in order to correct for any changes that might be due to growth of the kidney during the postnatal period.

Abstracted from Horster, M., and Valtin, H. *J. Clin. Invest.* 50:779, 1971.

Problem 5-2

The Clearance of Substances Having a Reabsorptive or a Secretory Tm. Micropuncture evidence that inulin is neither reabsorbed nor secreted by renal tubules was adduced only in recent years (Chap. 3). Until this direct proof became available, nephrologists relied on indirect evidence to validate inulin as a substance that can be used to measure the GFR. One important such line of evidence lay in the differences between the inulin clearance and the clearances of substances having a reabsorptive or secretory Tm.

We have previously established the following points: (a) that the formula for the renal clearance of any substance is $U \cdot \dot{V}/P$; (b) that $U \cdot \dot{V}$ gives the renal excretion of a substance; (c) that the inulin clearance is independent of the plasma concentration of inulin because the urinary excretion of inulin increases in direct proportion to the rise in plasma inulin concentration (see Problem 3-1 and the corresponding Answer); but (d) that the urinary excretion rates for substances having a reabsorptive Tm (e.g., phosphate or glucose, Fig. 4-1 and 4-3) or a secretory Tm (e.g., PAH, Fig. 5-1) vary curvilinearly as the plasma concentrations of such substances are changed. The last point tells us that, unlike the inulin clearance, the clearance of substances having transport maxima must vary as the plasma concentration of these substances is changed.

On a single graph, draw the general curves describing the clearance of inulin, glucose, and PAH as a function of increasing plasma concentrations of inulin, glucose, and PAH, respectively. Plot plasma concentrations on the abscissa against clearances on the ordinate.

Selected References

The Process of Secretion

Bayliss, L. E. The Process of Secretion. In F. R. Winton (Ed.), *Modern Views on the Secretion of Urine.* Churchill, London, 1956.

Chambers, R., and Kempton, R. T. Indications of function of the chick mesonephros in tissue culture with phenol red. *J. Cell. Comp. Physiol.* 3:131, 1933.

Cross, R. J., and Taggart, J. V. Renal tubular transport: Accumulation of p-aminohippurate by rabbit kidney slices. *Amer. J. Physiol.* 161:181, 1950.

Cushny, A. R. *The Secretion of the Urine.* Longmans, Green, London, 1917.

Forster, R. P. Active cellular transport of urea by the frog renal tubules. *Amer. J. Physiol.* 179:372, 1954.

Forster, R. P. Urea and the Early History of Renal Clearance Studies. In B. Schmidt-Nielsen (Ed.), *Urea and the Kidney.* Excerpta Medica Foundation, Amsterdam, 1970.

Marshall, E. K., Jr., and Crane, M. The secretory function of the renal tubules. *Amer. J. Physiol.* 70:465, 1924.

Marshall, E. K., Jr., and Grafflin, A. L. The structure and function of the kidney of *Lophius piscatorius. Bull. Johns Hopkins Hosp.* 43:205, 1928.

Marshall, E. K., Jr., and Vickers, J. L. The mechanism of the elimination of phenolsulphonphthalein by the kidney: A proof of secretion by the convoluted tubules. *Bull. Johns Hopkins Hosp.* 34:1, 1923.

Mudge, G. H., and Taggart, J. V. Effect of acetate on the renal excretion of p-aminohippurate in the dog. *Amer. J. Physiol.* 161:191, 1950.

Pitts, R. F. *Physiology of the Kidney and Body Fluids*, 2d ed. Year Book, Chicago, 1968. Chap. 8.

Shannon, J. A. The renal excretion of phenol red by the aglomerular fishes, *Opsanus tau* and *Lophius piscatorius. J. Cell. Comp. Physiol.* 11:315, 1938.

Shannon, J. A. Renal tubular excretion. *Physiol. Rev.* 19:63, 1939.

Smith, H. W. *Newer Methods of Study of Renal Function in Man.* Porter Lectures, Series IX. University Extension Division, University of Kansas, Lawrence, 1943.

Smith, H. W. *The Kidney: Structure and Function in Health and Disease.* Oxford University Press, New York, 1951.

Organic Acids and Bases

Berndt, W. O., and Grote, D. The accumulation of C^{14}-dinitrophenol by slices of rabbit kidney cortex. *J. Pharmacol. Exp. Ther.* 164:223, 1968.

Berndt, W. O. In vitro accumulation of ^{14}C-xanthine by rabbit renal cortex and its relationship to overall oxypurine transport. *Nephron* 7:339, 1970.

Beyer, K. H., Peters, L., Woodward, R., and Verwey, W. F. The enhancement of the physiological economy of penicillin in dogs by the simultaneous administration of para-aminohippuric acid. *J. Pharmacol. Exp. Ther.* 82:310, 1944.

Beyer, K. H., Russo, H. F., Tillson, E. K., Miller, A. K., Verwey, W. F., and Gass, S. R. Benemid, p-(di-n-propylsulfamyl)-

benzoic acid: Its renal affinity and its elimination. *Amer. J. Physiol.* 166:625, 1951.

Cohen, J. J., Chesney, R. W., Brand, P. H., Neville, H. F., and Blanchard, C. F. α-Ketoglutarate metabolism and K⁺ uptake by dog kidney slices. *Amer. J. Physiol.* 217:161, 1969.

Cohen, J. J., and Wittmann, E. Renal utilization and excretion of α-ketoglutarate in dog: Effect of alkalosis. *Amer. J. Physiol.* 204:795, 1963.

Forster, R. P., and Copenhaver, J. H., Jr. Intracellular accumulation as an active process in a mammalian renal transport system *in vitro:* Energy dependence and competitive phenomena. *Amer. J. Physiol.* 186:167, 1956.

Mudge, G. H., and Taggart, J. V. Effect of 2,4-dinitrophenol on renal transport mechanisms in the dog. *Amer. J. Physiol.* 161:173, 1950.

Selleck, B. H., and Cohen, J. J. Specific localization of α-ketoglutarate uptake to dog kidney and liver *in vivo. Amer. J. Physiol.* 208:24, 1965.

Sperber, I. Secretion of organic anions in the formation of urine and bile. *Pharmacol. Rev.* 11:109, 1959.

Taggart, J. V., and Forster, R. P. Renal tubular transport: Effect of 2,4-dinitrophenol and related compounds on phenol red transport in the isolated tubules of the flounder. *Amer. J. Physiol.* 161:167, 1950.

Weiner, I. M. Transport of Weak Acids and Bases. In J. Orloff and R. W. Berliner (Eds.), *Handbook of Physiology.* Section 8: Renal Physiology. American Physiological Society, Washington, D.C., 1973.

Weiner, I. M., and Mudge, G. H. Renal tubular mechanisms for excretion of organic acids and bases. *Amer. J. Med.* 36:743, 1964.

Renal Plasma Flow, Renal Blood Flow, Extraction

Horster, M., and Lewy, J. E. Filtration fraction and extraction of PAH during the neonatal period in the rat. *Amer. J. Physiol.* 219:1061, 1970.

Horster, M., and Valtin, H. Postnatal development of renal function: Micropuncture and clearance studies in the dog. *J. Clin. Invest.* 50:779, 1971.

Pilkington, L. A., Binder, R., de Haas, J. C. M., and Pitts, R. F. Intrarenal distribution of blood flow. *Amer. J. Physiol.* 208:1107, 1965.

Reubi, F. Objections à la théorie de la séparation intrarénale des hématies et du plasma (Pappenheimer). *Helv. Med. Acta* 25:516, 1958.

Smith, H. W. *The Renal Blood Flow in Normal Subjects.* Porter Lectures, Series IX. University Extension Division, University of Kansas, Lawrence, 1943.

Smith, H. W. *The Kidney: Structure and Function in Health and Disease.* Oxford University Press, New York, 1951.

6 : Renal Hemodynamics and Oxygen Consumption

The two kidneys of adult man together weigh about 300 g, and thus constitute less than 0.5% of the body weight. Yet, they are perfused by an amount of blood that is equal to 20 to 25% of the cardiac output, i.e., in excess of 1,000 ml per minute. The reason for this very high rate of perfusion is probably related to the evolutionary development of an organ with a high filtering capacity, as discussed in Chapter 1.

In addition to the high rate of flow, the renal circulation has a number of other characteristic features, some of which are unique. This chapter will concentrate on these features.

Hydrostatic Pressures and Resistances in the Renal Vascular Tree

Hydrostatic pressures in the major renal vessels are shown in Figure 6-1. The data shown are from rats, which are thus far the only mammals from which direct measurements of hydrostatic pressure in glomerular capillaries have been obtained. Although absolute values in man might be slightly different, the profile is almost certainly similar. Of particular importance are the large decreases in pressure that occur in the afferent and efferent arterioles, identifying these two vessels as the major sites of vascular resistance. Changes in the resistance within either of these vessels will alter the renal blood flow (RBF); but it is the differential changes in the resistances within both vessels that will determine the hydrostatic pressure within the glomerular capillaries, and hence the rate of glomerular ultrafiltration (see Fig. 3-1).

It is possible that the afferent and efferent arterioles of superficial cortical nephrons have different properties from the corresponding vessels of juxtamedullary nephrons. For example, efferent arterioles of juxtamedullary nephrons are surrounded by smooth muscles that appear to have cholinergic innervation; this may not be so for efferent arterioles arising from superficial cortical nephrons. Such differences could partly account for the

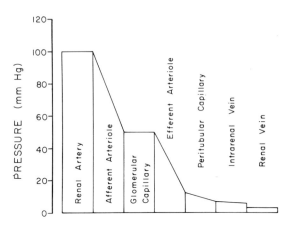

Figure 6-1
Hydrostatic pressure profile in the renal vascular tree of the rat. Data from Brenner, B. M., Troy, J. L., and Daugharty, T. M. *J. Clin. Invest.* 50:1776, 1971; and Proceedings of the XXV International Congress of Physiological Sciences, Abstract No. 229.

differential behavior of the renal circulation in different regions of the kidney, which are described below.

Intrarenal Differences in Glomerular Filtration

Two types of nephron, the superficial cortical and the juxta-medullary, were described in Chapter 1. Besides having anatomical distinctions, these nephrons also differ functionally. As shown in Table 6-1, under control conditions the so-called *single glomerular filtration rate* (gfr, as distinct from GFR, which refers to the glomerular filtration rate of the entire kidney) of a juxtamedullary nephron is greater than that of a nephron lying in more superficial parts of the cortex. Furthermore, differential changes in these filtration rates occur during various conditions. Water diuresis (defined in Chap. 7) is accompanied by a reduction in the gfr of juxtamedullary nephrons but no change in that of superficial cortical nephrons. An increase in sodium intake, on the other hand, is associated with an increase in the gfr of superficial cortical nephrons.

The functional significance of these changes is not yet clear; it is possible that they involve the regulation of sodium and water

Table 6-1
Intrarenal differences in the glomerular filtration rates of single nephrons
(gfr) of rats, under varying conditions.

Condition	Superficial Cortical Nephron (nanoliters/min)	Juxtamedullary Nephron (nanoliters/min)
Control (ADH present)[a]	30	50
Water diuresis (ADH absent)	30	35
High sodium intake	40	50

[a]ADH = antidiuretic hormone (see Chap. 8).

Note: All values are approximations that have been rounded off. They have been taken from the following: Horster, M., and Thurau, K. *Pflügers Arch. Ges. Physiol.* 301:162, 1968; Jamison, R. L. *Amer. J. Physiol.* 218:46, 1969; deRouffignac, C., Deiss, S., and Bonvalet, J. P. *Pflügers Eur. J. Physiol.* 315:273, 1970; Davis, J. M., and Schnermann, J. *Pflügers Eur. J. Physiol.* 330:323, 1971; Daugharty, T. M., Troy, J. L., and Brenner, B. M. Proceedings of the XXV International Congress of Physiological Sciences, Abstract No. 383.

balance (Chaps. 7 and 8). Nor have the mechanisms responsible for these changes been identified. The fact that the gfr of juxtamedullary nephrons is higher in the control state than during water diuresis must reflect a relative increase in the resistance of the efferent as opposed to the afferent arteriole (Fig. 6-3). But whether this resistance results from the direct action of the antidiuretic hormone (ADH) on the smooth muscles of efferent arterioles, or from other effects, such as increased viscosity of the vasa recta blood, is not yet known.

Intrarenal Differences in Blood Flow

Control

The total renal blood flow can be measured by relatively direct techniques, as with an electromagnetic flow meter attached to the renal artery, or indirectly through application of the Fick principle (see Chap. 5). Other methods, however, must be used to detect differences in blood flow to the major regions of the kidney. Such methods are based, variously, on the fractional tissue uptake of dyes or radioactive markers, on filling of the renal vasculature with a silicone rubber compound, on dye dilution curves recorded by tiny detectors inserted into the renal tissue, or on the rate of washout of certain markers from the tissue. Results obtained in dogs by the last two techniques are summarized in Table 6-2; the situation is similar in man. More

Table 6-2
Distribution of total renal blood flow (RBF) in dogs under control conditions.

Region	RBF (ml per 100 g of kidney per min)	Proportion of Total Renal Blood Flow (%)
Cortex	340	93
Outer medulla	21	6
Papilla	2.5	0.7

Note: All values are averages taken from the work of: Kramer, K., et al. *Pflügers Arch. Ges. Physiol.* 270:251, 1960; Deetjen, P., et al. *Pflügers Arch. Ges. Physiol.* 279:281, 1964; and Thorburn, G. D., et al. *Circ. Res.* 13:290, 1963.

than 90% of the total renal blood flow perfuses the cortical region. Considering that about one-quarter of the cardiac output goes to the kidneys, this amounts to a perfusion rate per unit of cortical tissue that is more than 100 times higher than that of resting muscle. Only a very small portion of the total renal blood flow enters the medulla, with about 1% perfusing the papilla. Again, however, since total renal blood flow is so great, the absolute flow per unit of papillary tissue is about 15 times greater than that of resting muscle.

The high cortical perfusion rate is almost certainly related to the evolutionary development of the kidney as a filtering organ and not to its oxygen requirements. The relatively low medullary perfusion, in turn, is crucial to the important function of the kidneys to conserve water; this is considered in detail in Chapter 8.

The mechanisms that so strikingly decrease the medullary blood flow as compared to cortical flow have not been entirely identified. It seems clear, however, that they do not involve a decrease in the vascular volume per unit of renal tissue, which is roughly the same — 20% — in the cortex, medulla, and papilla. There is, rather, an increased resistance to flow; this resistance appears to lie in the descending vasa recta, and it may be related to their length; to the smooth muscles in their efferent arterioles and their innervation; and/or to other factors, such as increased viscosity of medullary blood.

Hemorrhage

The renal circulation is exquisitely sensitive to blood loss. Even relatively small hemorrhages, which do not decrease the systemic blood pressure, can result in striking decreases in the renal blood flow. Furthermore, the reduction affects primarily the superficial cortex. Figure 6-2 shows kidneys of dogs in which the vasculature had been outlined through the injection of a silicone rubber compound. In contrast to the control situation, when there is uniform filling of the vessels throughout the cortex, after hemorrhage there is a selective reduction in the blood flow to the superficial cortex and increased filling in the juxtamedullary and outer medullary regions. A similar change in the distribution of renal blood is seen in other conditions, such as heart or liver failure. The fact that this pattern is also seen when the renal sympathetic nerves are stimulated may be a clue to at least one of the mechanisms that may cause the change in distribution.

Antidiuretic Hormone (ADH)

Normally, this hormone is present in the blood; its effect on the renal blood flow has been tested by first removing ADH from the circulation and then restoring it, usually in the same animal. In the absence of ADH, i.e., in water diuresis, blood flow to the superficial cortex is increased over the control situation, flow in the juxtamedullary region and outer medulla is decreased, and that in the papilla is increased. These changes in the distribution of renal blood flow can be returned to that of the control state by administering ADH. These results have been interpreted to reflect a vasoconstrictor action of ADH.

Mechanisms Causing Changes in GFR and RBF

The examples cited above are only a few of many influences that can alter the GFR and the RBF. It is important to realize at this point not only that these two functions can change, but also that each may simultaneously undergo different alterations in various regions of the kidney, and that there may be divergent shifts in the filtration rate and blood flow. The last point is illustrated in Figure 6-3. In an anesthetized dog under control conditions, the

(a)

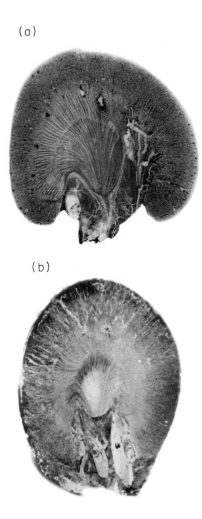

(b)

Figure 6-2
Sections of kidneys from dogs, during two conditions: (a) control and (b) after severe hemorrhage. The vasculature of both kidneys was filled with a silicone rubber compound at the same perfusion pressure. Note the even filling of all vessels, including the glomeruli, in the control animal. In contrast, there is selective reduction of blood flow to the superficial cortex during hemorrhage, reflecting increased resistance in this area. Increased filling of deeper areas reflects decreased resistance in the outer medulla. Photographs courtesy of A. C. Barger and R. Beeuwkes.

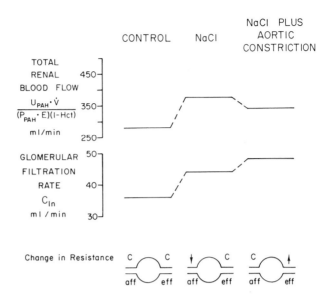

Figure 6-3
Changes in total renal blood flow (RBF) and glomerular filtration rate
(GFR) under varying conditions in a dog. Note that under some
circumstances, RBF and GFR will shift in the same direction, whereas
under other conditions they may undergo divergent changes. The variations
in resistance (C = control; ↓ = decrease; ↑ = increase) in the afferent and
efferent arterioles indicate the effect on the pressure gradient across the
glomeruli; these changes in gradient could be brought about by resistance
changes in one or both arterioles, and the diagrams merely indicate the
predominant alterations that must have occurred. The data on RBF and
GFR were abstracted from Earley, L. E. *Ann. N.Y. Acad. Sci.* 139:312,
1966.

RBF and GFR were found to be 280 and 36 ml per minute,
respectively. The resistances in the afferent and efferent arterioles
were presumably those of control conditions, designated by "C"
in the figure. When the dog was given an intravenous infusion of
NaCl, the RBF rose. Since the hydrostatic pressure in the renal
artery, the so-called renal perfusing pressure, did not change,
there must have been a decrease in resistance. The fact that the
GFR rose simultaneously means that this decrease in resistance
must have occurred proximal to the glomeruli, indicated in Figure
6-3 as a decrease in the resistance of the afferent arteriole. This is
not to exclude a simultaneous change in resistance in the efferent
arteriole; but the net effect must be a preponderant decrease
proximal to the glomerulus in order to account for the
concurrent increases in GFR and RBF. Mild constriction of the

aorta just above the renal artery reduced the renal perfusing pressure by 20 mm Hg. This caused a slight reduction of the RBF. The fact that it did not also decrease the GFR, but in fact increased it, must mean that the balance between afferent and efferent arteriolar resistances changed as if the resistance in the latter alone had increased. Such deductions, based on simultaneous changes in RBF and GFR, are also applied to locating the predominant site of resistance during autoregulation, which is discussed below.

With so many variables simultaneously influencing both the glomerular filtration rate and the blood flow, not only for the entire kidney but also for each nephron and depending on its location, it is perhaps not surprising that the mechanisms of control are not yet clear. Although normal renal function may be maintained after complete denervation, there is nevertheless evidence that the autonomic innervation of the kidneys has a functional role under some circumstances. There are also data that show the influence of humoral agents, such as ADH, the catecholamines, angiotensin, and the adrenal steroids. What is not yet clear, however, is on which vessel these factors exert their influence, in which region of the kidney, and under what circumstances.

Autoregulation of RBF and GFR

The phenomenon of autoregulation is illustrated in Figure 6-4, which portrays the RBF and the GFR measured simultaneously in dogs as their renal arterial pressure is varied. Note that over a range of pressure from about 80 to 180 mm Hg, a 100% increase in perfusing pressure causes an increase in RBF and GFR of less than 10%. This, by the formula $\dot{Q} = \dfrac{\Delta P}{R}$, must mean that somehow an increase in perfusing pressure is accompanied by a nearly equivalent increase in vascular resistance. By the deductions referred to in relation to Figure 6-3, the simultaneous "constancy" of GFR and RBF indicates that the predominant change in resistance must have occurred in the afferent arterioles.

Autoregulation persists even after complete renal denervation, after adrenal demedullation, and in a completely isolated kidney perfused in vitro. Hence, as the term is meant to indicate, autoregulation must be due to a change exclusively within the kidney, and brought about when the arterial perfusing pressure is altered.

Despite a great deal of work and the proposal of many theories, the mechanism of autoregulation has not been fully

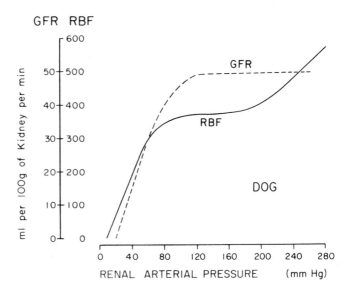

GFR RBF

Figure 6-4
Behavior of the renal blood flow (RBF) and glomerular filtration rate
(GFR) in dogs as the renal perfusing pressure is varied between 20 and 280
mm Hg. In the pressure range between about 80 and 180 mm Hg, both
RBF and GFR are autoregulated. Adapted from Shipley, R. E., and Study,
R. S. *Amer. J. Physiol.* 167:676, 1951.

identified. It seems likely that it involves smooth muscles in
afferent arterioles. One current theory states that an individual
nephron regulates itself through its juxtaglomerular apparatus
(JGA), which comprises the attachment of the early distal tubule
to the vascular pole of its own glomerulus (see Figs. 1-2 and 1-3).
The theory proposes that the load of sodium delivered to the
distal tubule is sensed by the JGA, which then adjusts the
resistance in the afferent arteriole, possibly by secreting renin and
converting it to angiotensin II; the greater the sodium load
delivered to the JGA, the lower the filtration rate in that nephron
(the gfr) and vice versa.

One interesting consequence of this hypothesis, should it turn
out to be correct, is that the biological reason for autoregulation
would not be the relative constancy of glomerular filtration and
renal blood flow per se, but rather of the filtered load of sodium.
That is, autoregulation of gfr would be a mechanism for adjusting
the tubular (i.e., filtered) load of sodium to the tubular capacity
for reabsorbing sodium; concomitant autoregulation of the blood
flow might then be a mere by-product of one mechanism by
which the kidneys maintain sodium balance (see Chap. 7).

Renal Oxygen
Consumption

According to the Fick principle, the oxygen consumption of an organ, $\dot{V}_{O_2}$, is related directly to the rate of blood flow to that organ, $\dot{Q}$, and to the difference in oxygen content between the artery, Ca_{O_2}, and vein, Cv_{O_2}, of that organ.

$$\dot{V}_{O_2} = \dot{Q}(Ca_{O_2} - Cv_{O_2}) \tag{6-1}$$

In most organs, such as skeletal muscle, the resting oxygen consumption remains constant as the blood flow to that organ is reduced. Consequently, the arteriovenous (a-v) oxygen content difference rises in proportion to the decrease in flow (Eq. 6-1). The heart is an exception, since even at rest the coronary a-v oxygen difference is very high, about 7 Vol%. Therefore, when coronary blood flow decreases, the oxygen supply to the myocardium is deficient. For this reason, the heart is known as a flow-limited organ.

There are two seeming paradoxes in renal oxygen consumption. (1) Even though this consumption per weight of renal tissue is greater than that of any other organ, the renal a-v oxygen difference is only about 1.7 Vol%, probably the lowest of any organ. (2) Despite the very low a-v oxygen difference, the kidneys behave like flow-limited organs. The solution to these paradoxes is illustrated in Figure 6-5; it involves the fact that the main renal requirement for oxidative energy is the tubular reabsorption of sodium.

As is shown in Figure 6-5a, as renal blood flow decreases from about 700 to 200 ml per 100 g of kidney per minute, the oxygen consumption decreases proportionally, so that the a-v oxygen difference does not change; that is, in these ranges of blood flow, the kidneys act like flow-limited organs. Only at very low rates of renal blood flow do the kidneys behave like most other organs, i.e., by extracting more oxygen from each unit of blood flowing through them.

The relationships shown in Figure 6-5a puzzled renal physiologists until it became clear that the true independent variable is not the renal blood flow but rather the glomerular filtration rate and hence the amount of sodium that is filtered ($P_{Na} \cdot GFR$). As is shown in Figure 6-5b, there is a direct correlation between the filtration rate and the oxygen consumption. With a relatively stable plasma sodium concentration (P_{Na}), the amount of sodium filtered into the tubular system varies in direct proportion to the GFR. And since virtually all the filtered sodium is reabsorbed, the true independent variable that determines renal oxygen con-

sumption is the amount of sodium that must be reabsorbed. This
fact is illustrated in Figure 6-5c, which is based on experiments
that showed a linear correlation between renal oxygen consumption and sodium reabsorption as the latter was varied by a
number of maneuvers.

When GFR, and hence sodium reabsorption, cease (Fig. 6-5b
and c), the remaining oxygen consumption reflects the basal
requirements of the renal tissue, which amounts to about
one-fifth of the total oxygen consumption of the normally
functioning kidney. Interestingly, this basal consumption of a
little less than 100 μMoles per 100 g of kidney per minute is
about the same as that of other epithelial tissues. It is only in this
range of oxygen requirements that the kidneys act like many
other organs, i.e., by extracting more oxygen when the rate of
flow is insufficient to meet the minimal needs.

Sodium reabsorption is an active process (see Chap. 7) which,
according to the direct correlation shown in Figure 6-5c, depends
largely on energy derived from oxidative metabolism. This
deduction fits well with the fact that most of the filtered sodium
is reabsorbed in the proximal and distal tubules (see Fig. 7-7), i.e.,
in the renal cortex, which undergoes mainly aerobic metabolism;
in contrast, renal medullary structures derive much energy from
anaerobic metabolism. The cost of reabsorbing filtered sodium is
about 1 μMole of oxygen for every 28 μEq of sodium reabsorbed

Summary

The mammalian renal circulation has a number of unique
features. Per unit of tissue weight, the kidneys are perfused by
more blood and they consume more oxygen than almost any
other organ. Yet, the renal arteriovenous (a-v) oxygen content
difference is lower than that of other organs. The rate of renal
blood flow (RBF) and the filtration rate of individual glomeruli
(gfr) vary not only under different conditions but also in
different regions of the kidney. Ordinarily, both variables are
autoregulated in most nephrons.

These unique features are best understood in the context of
salt and water balance. Probably through evolutionary forces, the
kidney became an organ of high filtering capacity. As a necessary
concomitant, the RBF is far in excess of the basal oxygen
requirements, so that the a-v oxygen content difference is very
low. In most terrestrial mammals, the potential liability of high
filtration is counteracted by virtually complete reabsorption of
the filtered water and sodium. The latter requires energy (see
Chap. 7) and is, in fact, the process that accounts for the high

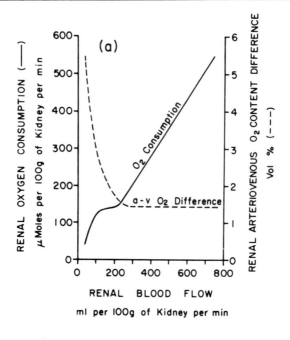

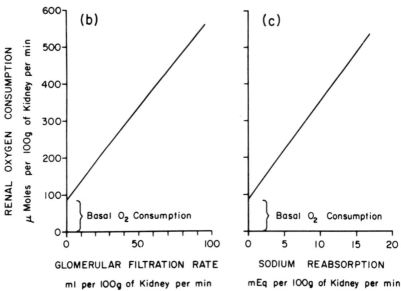

Figure 6-5
Experiments in dogs, which solved the puzzle that even though oxygen consumption is very high per unit of renal tissue, the renal arteriovenous (a-v) oxygen content difference is very low; and that despite the low a-v oxygen content difference, the kidneys act like flow-limited organs over a wide range of renal blood flow.

(a) As renal blood flow decreases to about 200 ml per 100 g of kidney per minute, renal oxygen consumption decreases proportionally, so that the a-v oxygen content difference does not change

rate of renal oxygen consumption. But since an increased rate of filtration is ordinarily accompanied by an increase in the RBF, the greater need for oxygen is "automatically" met so that an increase in oxygen extraction is not required. Similarly, the raison d'etre for autoregulation may well be the regulation of sodium excretion through adjustment of the glomerular filtration rate, with regulation of the blood flow being a coincidental event. Finally, the intrarenal distribution of the blood flow and filtration rate may also be governed primarily by the need for the conservation of sodium and water.

Selected References

General

Barger, A. C., and Herd, J. A. The renal circulation. *New Eng. J. Med.* 284:482, 1971.

Barger, A. C., and Herd, J. A. Renal Vascular Anatomy and Distribution of Blood Flow. In J. Orloff and R. W. Berliner (Eds.), *Handbook of Physiology.* Section 8: Renal Physiology. American Physiological Society, Washington, D.C., 1973.

Brenner, B. M., Troy, J., MacInnes, R., and Daugharty, T. Direct assessment of pressures, flows, and resistances across single glomerular units of the rat kidney. *J. Clin. Invest.* 51:14a, 1972.

Fourman, J., and Moffat, D. B. *The Blood Vessels of the Kidney.* Blackwell, Oxford, 1971.

Kiil, F. Blood Flow and Oxygen Utilization by the Kidney. In J. W. Fisher (Ed.), *Kidney Hormones.* Academic, New York, 1971.

(Eq. 6-1). In these experiments, the changes in renal blood flow were either spontaneous or induced by altering renal perfusing pressure after autoregulation had been abolished.

(b) In these experiments, the glomerular filtration rate (GFR) varied directly as the renal blood flow. The relationship between the filtration rate and renal oxygen consumption was linear over the entire range of GFR. Since plasma sodium concentration did not change, the rate at which sodium was filtered ($P_{Na} \cdot$ GFR) must have varied in direct proportion to the GFR, suggesting that the oxidative energy required to reabsorb sodium might be the true independent variable that determines the rate of renal oxygen consumption.

(c) This suggestion was confirmed by varying the rate of renal sodium reabsorption by means other than, and in addition to, changes in GFR. The experimental maneuvers included constriction of the renal vein, and intravenous infusions of Na^+ salts. No matter how sodium reabsorption was varied, oxygen consumption changed proportionately.

These graphs are based on data from the following references: Kramer, K., and Deetjen, P. *Pflügers Arch. Ges. Physiol.* 271:782, 1960; Lassen, N. A., Munck, O., and Thaysen, J. H. *Acta Physiol. Scand.* 51:371, 1961; Deetjen, P., and Kramer, K. *Pflügers Arch. Ges. Physiol.* 273:636, 1961.

Selkurt, E. E. The Renal Circulation. In W. F. Hamilton and P. Dow (Eds.), *Handbook of Physiology.* Section 2: Circulation, vol. II. American Physiological Society, Washington, D.C., 1963.

Sherwood, T., and Lavender, J. P. Renal medullary perfusion: Direct observations by fine detail angiography in the dog. *Nephron* 8:317, 1971.

Smith, H. W. *Physiology of the Renal Circulation.* The Harvey Lectures, 1939—1940. Science Press, Lancaster, 1940.

Thurau, K., and Levine, D. Z. The Renal Circulation. In C. Rouiller and A. F. Muller (Eds.), *The Kidney,* vol. III. Academic, New York, 1971.

Trueta, J., Barclay, A. E., Daniel, P. M., Franklin, K. J., and Prichard, M. M. C. *Studies of the Renal Circulation.* Blackwell, Oxford, 1948.

Winton, F. R. Present concepts of the renal circulation. *Arch. Intern. Med.* (Chicago) 103:495, 1959.

Methods

de Rouffignac, C., Deiss, S., and Bonvalet, J. P. Détermination du taux individuel de filtration glomérulaire des néphrons accessibles et inaccessibles à la microponction. *Pflügers Eur. J. Physiol.* 315:273, 1970.

Fourman, J., and Moffat, D. B. *The Blood Vessels of the Kidney.* Blackwell, Oxford, 1971.

Hanssen, O. D. The relationship between glomerular filtration and length of the proximal convoluted tubules in mice. *Acta Pathol. Microbiol. Scand.* 53:265, 1961.

Kramer, K., Thurau, K., and Deetjen, P. Hämodynamik des Nierenmarks: I. Mitteilung. Capilläre Passagezeit, Blutvolumen, Durchblutung, Gewebshämatokrit und O_2-Verbrauch des Nierenmarks in situ. *Pflügers Arch. Ges. Physiol.* 270:251, 1960.

Smith, H. W. *The Kidney: Structure and Function in Health and Disease.* Oxford University Press, New York, 1951.

Thurau, K. Renal hemodynamics. *Amer. J. Med.* 36:698, 1964.

Thorburn, G. D., Kopald, H. H., Herd, J. A., Hollenberg, M., O'Morchoe, C. C. C., and Barger, A. C. Intrarenal distribution of nutrient blood flow determined with Krypton 85 in the unanesthetized dog. *Circ. Res.* 13:290, 1963.

Wright, F. S., and Giebisch, G. Glomerular filtration in single nephrons. *Kidney Int.* 1:201, 1972.

Intrarenal Distribution of Blood Flow and Glomerular Filtration

Carriere, S., Thorburn, G. D., O'Morchoe, C. C. C., and Barger, A. C. Intrarenal distribution of blood flow in dogs during haemorrhagic hypotension. *Circ. Res.* 19:167, 1966.

Davis, J. M., and Schnermann, J. The effect of antidiuretic hormone on the distribution of nephron filtration rates in rats with hereditary diabetes insipidus. *Pflügers Eur. J. Physiol.* 330:323, 1971.

Fisher, R. D., Grunfeld, J. P., and Barger, A. C. Intrarenal distribution of blood flow in diabetes insipidus: Role of ADH. *Amer. J. Physiol.* 219:1348, 1970.

Horster, M., and Thurau, K. Micropuncture studies on the filtration rate of single superficial and juxtamedullary glomeruli in the rat kidney. *Pflügers Arch. Ges. Physiol.* 301:162, 1968.

Kew, M. C., Varma, R. R., Williams, H. S., Brunt, P. W., Hourigan, K. J., and Sherlock, S. Renal and intrarenal blood-flow in cirrhosis of the liver. *Lancet* 2:504, 1971.

Ladefoged, J., and Munck, O. Distribution of Blood Flow in the Kidney. In J. W. Fisher (Ed.), *Kidney Hormones.* Academic, New York, 1971.

Norvell, J. E. Renal nerves: Are they essential? *New Eng. J. Med.* 283:261, 1970.

Pomeranz, B. H., Birtch, A. G., and Barger, A. C. Neural control of intrarenal blood flow. *Amer. J. Physiol.* 215:1067, 1968.

Autoregulation

Assaykeen, T. A. (Ed.). *Control of Renin Secretion.* Advances in Experimental Medicine and Biology, vol. XVII. Plenum, New York, 1972.

Cook, W. F. Cellular Localization of Renin. In J. W. Fisher (Ed.), *Kidney Hormones.* Academic, New York, 1971.

Forster, R. P., and Maes, J. P. Effects of experimental neurogenic hypertension on renal blood flow and glomerular filtration rates in intact denervated kidneys of unanesthetized rabbits with adrenal glands demedullated. *Amer. J. Physiol.* 150:534, 1947.

Goormaghtigh, N. Existence of an endocrine gland in the media of the renal arterioles. *Proc. Soc. Exper. Biol. Med.* 42:688, 1939.

Granger, P., Dahlheim, H., and Thurau, K. Enzyme activities of the single juxtaglomerular apparatus in the rat kidney. *Kidney Int.* 1:78, 1972.

Gross, F. Renin Stores in the Kidney and Plasma Renin Activity. In J. W. Fisher (Ed.), *Kidney Hormones.* Academic, New York, 1971.

Johnson, P. C. (Ed.). Autoregulation of blood flow. *Circ. Res.* 15:I-1, 1964. Section 4 of this symposium presents the various theories for the mechanism of autoregulation of the renal blood flow and glomerular filtration rate.

Thurau, K., Schnermann, J., Nagel, W., Horster, M., and Wahl, M. Composition of tubular fluid in the macula densa segment as a factor regulating the function of the juxtaglomerular apparatus. *Circ. Res.* 21(Suppl. 2):79, 1967.

Tobian, L. Physiology of the juxtaglomerular cells. *Ann. Intern. Med.* 52:395, 1960.

Vander, A. J. Control of renin release. *Physiol. Rev.* 47:359, 1967.

Renal
Metabolism

Abodeely, D. A., and Lee, J. B. Fuel of respiration of outer renal medulla. *Amer. J. Physiol.* 220:1693, 1971.

Cohen, J. J., and Barac-Nieto, M. Renal Metabolism of Substrates in Relation to Renal Function. In J. Orloff and R. W. Berliner (Eds.), *Handbook of Physiology.* Section 8: Renal Physiology. American Physiological Society, Washington, D.C., 1973.

Deetjen, P. Normal and Critical Oxygen Supply of the Kidney. In D. W. Lubbers, U. C. Luft, G. Thews, and E. Witzleb (Eds.), *Oxygen Transport in Blood and Tissue.* Thieme, Stuttgart, 1968.

Deetjen, P., and Kramer, K. Die Abhängigkeit des O_2-Verbrauchs der Niere von der Na-Rückresorption. *Pflügers Arch. Ges. Physiol.* 273:636, 1961.

Kiil, F., Aukland, K., and Refsum, H. E. Renal sodium transport and oxygen consumption. *Amer. J. Physiol.* 201:511, 1961.

Krebs, H. A. Renal Carbohydrate and Fatty Acid Metabolism. In K. Thurau and H. Jahrmärker (Eds.), *Renal Transport and Diuretics.* Springer, New York, 1969.

Lassen, N. A., Munck, O., and Thaysen, J. H. Oxygen consumption and sodium reabsorption in the kidney. *Acta Physiol. Scand.* 51:371, 1961.

Lee, J. B., and Peter, H. M. Effect of oxygen tension on glucose metabolism in rabbit kidney cortex and medulla. *Amer. J. Physiol.* 217:1464, 1969.

Lymph Flow   Bell, R. D., Keyl, M. J., Shrader, F. R., Jones, E. W., and Henry, L. P. Renal lymphatics: The internal distribution. *Nephron* 5:454, 1968.

Kriz, W., and Dieterich, H. J. Das Lymphgefäss-system der Niere bei einigen Säugetieren. Licht- und elektronenmikroskopische Untersuchungen. *Z. Anat. Entwicklungsgesch.* 131:111, 1970.

LeBrie, S. J. Renal lymph and osmotic diuresis. *Amer. J. Physiol.* 215:116, 1968.

LeBrie, S. J., and Mayerson, H. S. Influence of elevated venous pressure on flow and composition of renal lymph. *Amer. J. Physiol.* 198:1037, 1960.

Mayerson, H. S. The Physiologic Importance of Lymph. In W. F. Hamilton and P. Dow (Eds.), *Handbook of Physiology.* Section 2: Circulation, vol. II. American Physiological Society, Washington, D.C., 1963.

Yoffey, J. M., and Courtice, F. C. Lymph Flow from Regional Lymphatics. In *Lymphatics, Lymph and the Lymphomyeloid Complex.* Academic, New York, 1970.

7 : Na⁺ and H₂O Transport. Na⁺ Balance

Definitions

The following definitions conform to the common usage of the terms in renal physiology.

Diuresis: urine flow that is greater than normal, i.e., in excess of about 1 ml per minute in adult man.

Osmotic diuresis: increased urine flow that is due to extra amount of nonreabsorbed solute within the tubular lumen. A common example is mannitol diuresis.

Water diuresis: increased urine flow that is due to decreased reabsorption of "free" (i.e., solute-free) water. This type of diuresis is seen in persons who have drunk large amounts of dilute fluid (see Problem 8-1 and the corresponding Answer) and in patients with diabetes insipidus, who have some abnormality of the antidiuretic hormone (ADH or vasopressin).

Antidiuresis: urine flow that is less than normal, usually below about 0.5 ml per minute in adult man. The term is also frequently used to connote the excretion of urine that is hyperosmotic to plasma.

Osmolality: the concentration of discrete — i.e., osmotically active — particles in solution. Osmolality is a function of the number of particles in solution, regardless of their mass, charge, or size. The common units in biological fluids are milliosmoles per kilogram of H_2O (mOsm/kg H_2O).

Isosmotic: equal to the osmolality of plasma, which normally is about 290 mOsm/kg H_2O. Because it is a round figure that is easy to remember, 300 mOsm/kg H_2O is frequently used for plasma.

The term is also used to connote equality with the osmolality of any other solution, be that more or less concentrated than plasma; e.g., isosmotic absorption by the gallbladder refers to the reabsorbate having the same osmolality as the luminal fluid. This additional meaning is sometimes also applied to "hyperosmotic" and "hyposmotic."

Hyperosmotic: greater than the osmolality of plasma. Maximally concentrated human urine has an osmolality of about

1,200 mOsm/kg H_2O at the same time that plasma osmolality remains around 300 mOsm/kg H_2O.

Hyposmotic: less than the osmolality of plasma. Maximally dilute human urine has an osmolality of about 50 mOsm/kg H_2O at the same time that plasma osmolality remains around 300 mOsm/kg H_2O.

Correlation of Na+ and H₂O Transport

The balance of Na^+ and H_2O depends critically on these substances being avidly reabsorbed by the renal tubules (see Table 1-1). Water reabsorption by renal tubules (and in fact all epithelial membranes) is a passive process that depends upon osmotic gradients between the tubular lumen and some site within the tubular epithelium. Normally, Na^+ (and mainly Cl^-) are the most abundant osmotically active particles in tubular fluid. Hence, water diffuses passively in response to an osmotic gradient set up by Na^+ (and Cl^-).

Na+ and H₂O Reabsorption in Proximal Tubules

Early micropuncture experiments showed that fluid reabsorbed from the proximal tubule was isosmotic; that is, even after two-thirds of the fluid that was filtered had been reabsorbed, the fluid remaining within the proximal tubular lumen had the same osmolality as plasma (Fig. 7-3); the concentrations of Na^+ (and under some conditions, of Cl^-) in this tubular fluid were also identical with those in plasma. These findings could be interpreted as reflecting reabsorption of water as the initial event, followed secondarily by reabsorption of NaCl; or conversely, the primary event could have been reabsorption of NaCl, followed by water. The experiment illustrated in Figure 7-1 showed that the latter alternative is correct.

Na+ Reabsorption Is Primary and Active

The experiment was performed on the proximal tubule of *Necturus;* the important results have been confirmed in proximal and distal tubules of mammalian species, only some specific numerical values being different. The rationale of the experiment was that if the primary reabsorption of water initiated the reabsorption of NaCl, net flux of water should be independent of the intratubular concentration of NaCl; but if the converse were the case — i.e., if water reabsorption followed that of NaCl, and if, furthermore, the reabsorption of NaCl depended in part on its concentration in tubular fluid — there should be a correlation between the intratubular concentration of NaCl and the net flux of water.

Figure 7-1a illustrates the technique of stop-flow micro-perfusion. In Step (1), the early part of the proximal tubule is filled with oil. By means of a micropipet inserted into the middle of the oil column, the tubular lumen is then filled with solution, thereby splitting the column of oil (Step 2). The solution, which has different concentrations of NaCl, is left within the tubular lumen until a steady concentration of NaCl has been attained. The time interval required to reach a steady concentration is 20 minutes in *Necturus* and about 30 seconds in rats. The fluid is then withdrawn through a third micropipet that is inserted into the distal end of the stationary fluid column (Step 3). The injected fluid column (Step 2) contains NaCl at varying concentrations, trace amounts of inulin, and enough mannitol to render the fluid isosmotic with plasma.

The results of such an experiment in the proximal tubule of *Necturus* are shown in Figure 7-1b. Net flux of water could be calculated from the inulin concentration of the fluid that was withdrawn in Step (3) (see Chap. 3). At NaCl concentrations above 66 mMoles/liter, water was reabsorbed from the tubule, but at concentrations below this value, water entered the tubule. Clearly, then, the net flux of water is correlated with the intratubular concentration of NaCl, strongly arguing, by the rationale of the experiment, that movement of NaCl is the primary event.

This conclusion is supported by a further argument. Active transport of water by the kidney had been rejected earlier on the basis of thermodynamic arguments. Calculations suggested that the rate of expenditure of free energy that would be required to maintain observed differences in osmolality between plasma and hyperosmotic urine was about 1,000 times greater than the maximal rate for living cells. In fact, to date, active water transport has not been demonstrated in any biological system. Thus, the movement of water shown in Figure 7-1b was presumably passive, and since the experiment was so designed that no osmotic gradients existed between tubular fluid and interstitium when the fluid was first instilled, water movement could not have been primary.

Na⁺ Transport Against a Chemical Gradient. In the lower abscissa of Figure 7-1b, the intratubular concentration of NaCl has been expressed as milliequivalents of Na⁺ per liter. The Na⁺ concentration in plasma of *Necturus* is about 100 mEq/liter. Hence, in that portion of the experiment in which water moved

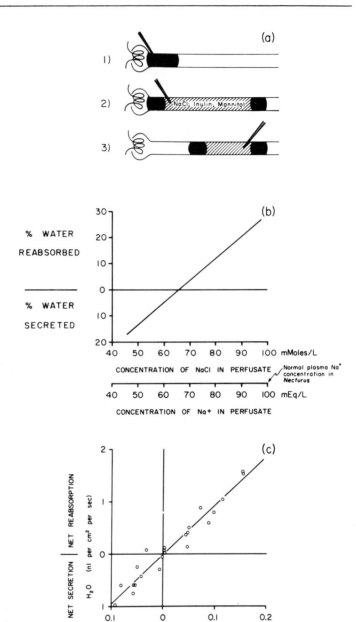

Figure 7-1

(a) Illustration of the technique of stop-flow microperfusion.

(b) Results of stop-flow microperfusion experiments in the proximal tubule of *Necturus*. Inasmuch as the net flux of NaCl in and out of the

out of the tubule (reflecting primary movement of NaCl), Na^+ must have been reabsorbed against a concentration gradient. At Na^+ concentrations below 66 mEq/liter, Na^+, and hence water, moved into the tubule. This has been interpreted to mean that the proximal tubular epithelium of *Necturus* cannot transport Na^+ against a concentration difference exceeding about 34 mEq/liter (the "limiting" concentration difference). When this maximal gradient is surpassed, there is net movement of Na^+ (and Cl^-) into the lumen, and water follows. The concentration of 66 mEq/liter is called the steady-state Na^+ concentration. In the proximal tubule of rats, this concentration has a value of about 107 mEq/liter. Since the plasma Na^+ concentration of rats is about 140 mEq/liter, the limiting concentration difference against which their proximal tubules can transport Na^+ is also in the range of 35 mEq/liter.

That NaCl did in fact move out of the tubule when water was reabsorbed, and into the tubule when water was secreted, is shown in Figure 7-1c. In the same experiment, as is shown in Figure 7-1a and b, net flux was calculated not only for water but also for solute, and the results demonstrate a direct and linear correlation between the net flux of solute and the net flux of water.

Na+ Transport Against an Electrical Potential Gradient. The experiment depicted in Figure 7-1 shows that movement of NaCl is the initial event, and that Na^+ is reabsorbed against a chemical concentration gradient. In order to determine whether the transport of Na^+ is active, one must in addition know the electrical potential differences (P.D.'s) across the proximal tubular cells. These are shown in Figure 7-2. Electrical P.D.'s were measured by inserting microelectrodes into the tubular lumen and into the cell, arbitrarily taking peritubular fluid as a zero reference. It is not yet certain whether in proximal tubules of mammals, the transepithelial P.D. (i.e., the P.D. between peri-

---

tubule depends in part on the intratubular concentration of NaCl, the direct relationship shown here strongly suggests that solute flux is primary and water follows passively. This point is further illustrated in part (c).

(c) Direct and linear correlation between net flux of solute and net flux of water in the same experiment. Since water moves passively in all biological systems that have been examined, and there were no initial osmotic gradients (Step 2), water must have moved secondarily in response to movement of solute.

Modified from: Shipp, J. C., et al. *Amer. J. Physiol.* 195:563, 1958; and Windhager, E. E., et al. *Amer. J. Physiol.* 197:313, 1959.

PROXIMAL TUBULE

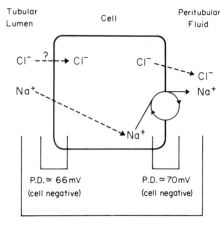

Figure 7-2
Electrical potential profile and transport of Na^+ and Cl^- across a mammalian proximal tubular cell. There is some disagreement whether a transepithelial electrical potential difference (P.D.) exists; however, resolution of this issue will not alter the conclusions that are presented in the text regarding the mode of Na^+ and Cl^- transport.

tubular fluid and tubular lumen) is zero or about 4 millivolts (mV) with the lumen being negative in respect to peritubular fluid; in *Necturus* it appears to be about 20 mV (lumen negative). For the sake of clarity, the value of 4 mV has been used in Figure 7-2. The P.D. between cell interior and peritubular fluid has a value of about 70 mV, the interior of the cell being negative to the peritubular fluid. The P.D. across the luminal membrane is then about 66 mV, the cell interior being negative in relation to the luminal fluid.

Since the intracellular Na^+ concentration is relatively low as compared to plasma (and hence to proximal tubular fluid), Na^+ movement from lumen into cell need not be active, but could proceed passively down an electrochemical potential gradient. This fact is expressed by the broken downward arrow. In its movement from cell interior to peritubular fluid and blood, however, Na^+ must be transported against an electrochemical potential gradient. Hence, this movement is indicated by a solid upward arrow involving an energy-consuming pump at the peritubular cell membrane. The negatively charged Cl ion has to move into the cell against an electrical gradient. Although the Cl^- concentration in luminal fluid exceeds that within the cell, the difference is not sufficiently large to overcome the electrical P.D. and permit passive diffusion of Cl^- into the cell. Nevertheless, entry of chloride into the cell may be passive, perhaps as neutral NaCl. The uncertainty regarding the mode of transport of Cl^- from lumen into cell is indicated by the broken arrow and question mark. Once in the cell, Cl^- can diffuse passively into the peritubular fluid, even against its chemical concentration gradient, since the electrical potential gradient favors its movement out of the cell.

Thus, the combined chemical and electrical analysis of the *SUMMARY* proximal tubule indicates that Na^+ is transported actively, and Cl^- perhaps passively; H_2O is reabsorbed passively as a consequence of the movement of NaCl.

Isosmotic Fluid Reabsorption

It has already been mentioned that the fluid that is reabsorbed from the proximal tubules is isosmotic with plasma. This fact, which is illustrated in Figure 7-3, is characteristic of Na^+ and water transport in many epithelial membranes, including, among others, the gallbladder; the ileum; and the secretion of gastric juice, pancreatic juice, and cerebrospinal fluid. The problem of so-called isosmotic fluid reabsorption can be illustrated for the mammalian proximal tubule. We have reviewed the evidence that water transport in the kidney, as in other biological systems, appears to be passive. From knowledge of the water permeability of the proximal tubule, it could be estimated that an osmotic gradient of about 23 mOsm/kg H_2O between tubular fluid and peritubular plasma would be required to account for the high rate of net water flux out of the tubule. Yet, as is shown in Figure 7-3, no such gradient could be demonstrated. Possible solutions to the problem were suggested independently by P. F. Curran and by J. M. Diamond, who proposed schemes in which the osmotic gradient is located within the epithelial structure itself. One possible scheme is illustrated in Figure 7-4.

Na^+ is actively transported from the cell into the lateral intercellular space, especially at the luminal end of the space. Membrane a has a high reflection coefficient for Na^+; i.e., its permeability for Na^+ is very low relative to the permeability for water. Consequently, Na^+ remains within the lateral intercellular space, and water flows passively into the space in response to the osmotic gradient. If the lateral intercellular channel is sufficiently

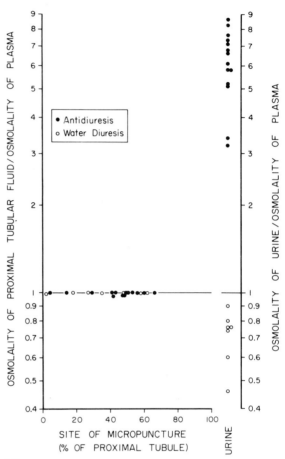

Figure 7-3

Results of micropunctures in rats, demonstrating isosmotic fluid reabsorption from the proximal tubules. Proximal tubular fluid has the same osmolality as plasma, whether the urine is more concentrated than plasma (antidiuresis) or less concentrated than plasma (water diuresis). The site of micropuncture was determined at the end of the experiment, through microdissection of the nephron. Only about the first 60% of the proximal tubule is accessible to micropuncture, since the last portion of the tubule dips beneath the surface of the kidney (see Fig. 1-2). Data from Gottschalk, C. W., and Mylle, M. *Amer. J. Physiol.* 196:927, 1959. The same type of results were obtained by A. M. Walker, P. A. Bott, J. Oliver, and M. C. MacDowell in some of the earliest renal micropuncture studies. *Amer. J. Physiol.* 134:580, 1941.

long and narrow, the fluid at the peritubular end of the channel will be osmotically equilibrated with the cellular fluid. Membrane β which might be the basement membrane or the capillary wall, is postulated to have a high hydraulic permeability to water, as

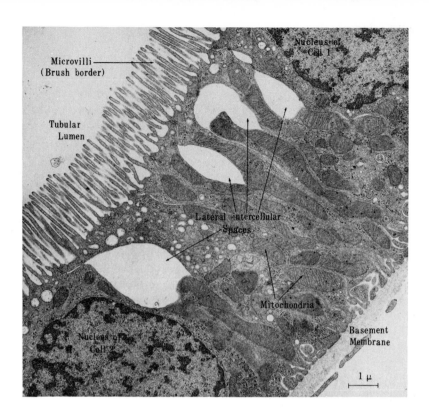

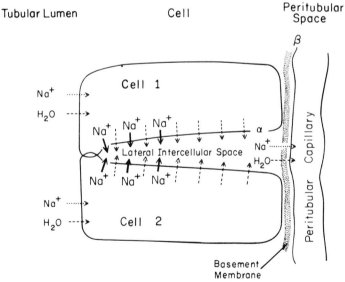

Figure 7-4

Postulated mechanism for isosmotic fluid transport by epithelial membranes. At the top is an electron micrograph of proximal tubular epithelium from a rat; it serves to orient the model at the bottom. The lateral intercellular spaces of the proximal tubular epithelium follow a serpentine course; hence it is seldom possible to portray a single intercellular channel extending from the apex to the base of a cell. Solid arrows = active Na^+ transport; dotted arrows = passive Na^+ transport; and interrupted arrows = passive water movement. Electron micrograph courtesy of C. C. Tisher.

opposed to membrane a, which has a low hydraulic permeability. Hence, as pressure builds up within the lateral intercellular space, there is bulk flow of isosmotic fluid preferentially across the basement membrane and into the peritubular capillary. Thus, this mechanism accomplishes net transfer of isosmotic fluid from tubular lumen to peritubular capillary; the driving osmotic gradient for the passive movement of water, which for so long eluded investigators, is postulated to be across the membrane lining the intercellular space. The Na^+ pump within this membrane is analogous to the pump within the peritubular membrane in Figure 7-2; in fact, the lateral intercellular space is visualized as an anatomical extension of the peritubular space.

Experimental support for this type of mechanism has recently been obtained. High rates of transepithelial water flux are associated with widening of the lateral intercellular spaces in a number of organs, including the kidney. This finding suggests that much of the water may traverse these spaces. Most importantly, hypertonicity of fluid within an intercellular channel — in this case, in an insect — has been demonstrated through direct micropuncture.

Na⁺ and H₂O Reabsorption in Other Nephron Segments

Loops of Henle

Thin Loops. Thin descending limbs of Henle may or may not have a slight transepithelial electrical P.D., of perhaps 3 mV, with the lumen being negative to the peritubular fluid. The transepithelial P.D. in ascending thin limbs is greater, about 10 mV, again with the lumen being negative. Electrical P.D.'s between cell interior and peritubular fluid have not yet been measured in thin loops of Henle, and it has not been definitely established whether chemical concentration gradients for Na^+ exist between tubular lumen and vasa recta plasma in either thin descending or thin ascending limbs. Some Na^+ may be secreted into the thin descending limbs, and this transport is passive. Almost certainly there is net reabsorption of Na^+ out of thin ascending limbs, but the mode of transport, whether active or passive, has not been settled. In the loops, water does not necessarily follow Na^+; it moves out of the thin descending limb, and is reabsorbed only slightly from the thin ascending limb. The mechanism and reasons for this divergence are considered in Chapter 8.

Thick Ascending Limbs. These structures lie deep within the renal medulla and hence are not accessible to direct analysis in vivo, as by micropuncture. Nevertheless, on the basis of indirect evidence, which is described in Chapter 8 (namely, low concentration of Na^+ and of Cl^-, and low osmolality of fluid in the early portion of the distal tubule), it seems certain that either Na^+ or Cl^- is reabsorbed actively from thick ascending limbs of Henle. Water, however, does not follow solute except in negligible amounts, presumably because the water permeability of the thick limbs is very low.

Distal Tubules   A distal tubular cell is presented in Figure 7-5. The transepithelial electrical P.D. is 30 to 60 mV, the latter value applying to the late portions of the distal tubule; the lumen is negative in respect to the peritubular fluid. The P.D. between peritubular fluid and cell interior also increases as a function of length along the distal tubule, from about 70 to 90 mV, with the intracellular fluid being negative in relation to the zero reference in peritubular fluid. The P.D. across the luminal membrane is about 20 to 40 mV, the cell interior being negative to the luminal fluid.

DISTAL TUBULE

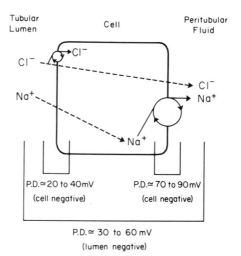

Figure 7-5
Electrical potential profile and transport of Na^+ and Cl^- across a mammalian distal tubular cell. The electrical potential differences (P.D.'s) increase as the later portions of the distal tubule are approached.

In analogy with the description for the proximal tubule (Fig. 7-2), Na^+ can diffuse passively down the electrochemical potential gradient from the lumen into the cell, but it must be transported actively against this gradient across the peritubular cell boundary. (As discussed in connection with Fig. 7-4, this boundary may in fact be the membrane lining the lateral intercellular spaces and basilar infoldings.) That distal tubular cells can transport Na^+ against an electrochemical potential gradient has been shown by stop-flow microperfusion experiments (Fig. 7-1). The steady-state Na^+ concentration (see p. 105) may be as low as 20 to 40 mEq/liter, indicating that distal tubular cells can transport Na^+ against a chemical concentration gradient of at least 100 mEq/liter (plasma Na^+ concentration in rats being about 140 mEq/liter). Cl^- can usually diffuse passively across both the luminal and peritubular cell membranes. In severe Cl^- deprivation, however, the concentration of Cl^- in the distal tubular fluid may be < 1.0 mEq/ liter. The Nernst equation shows that under these circumstances a transepithelial P.D. of 186 mV would be required for Cl^- reabsorption to be wholly passive; no P.D. of this magnitude has been recorded in any portion of the distal tubule. Thus, under certain circumstances, Cl^- reabsorption in the distal tubule may be active, and this possibility has been indicated in Figure 7-5 by the Cl^- "pump" at the luminal membrane.

The rate of water reabsorption from the distal tubules varies, depending on the concentration of the antidiuretic hormone (Chap. 8). In the presence of this hormone (vasopressin, or ADH), the rate of water reabsorption is high, whereas in the absence of ADH the rate is low.

Collecting Ducts

As is shown in Figure 7-6, the transepithelial electrical P.D. in collecting ducts varies, from about 60 to 16 mV, the lumen at all times being negative to the peritubular fluid. The P.D. declines along the length of the collecting duct, being highest in ducts lying in the cortex, and lowest near the tip of the papilla. It is possible that the low value is partly due to short-circuiting through the open end at the papillary tip. Potential differences between peritubular fluid and cell interior have not yet been measured in collecting ducts in vivo. Assuming these to be about 70 to 90 mV, as in the distal tubules, and assuming the P.D. across the luminal membrane to be as indicated in Figure 7-6, Na^+ could diffuse passively from lumen into cell under most conditions, but it must be pumped actively against an electro-

COLLECTING DUCT

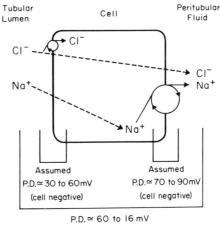

Figure 7-6
Electrical potential profile and transport of Na^+ and Cl^- across a mammalian collecting duct cell. The electrical potential differences (P.D.'s) across the luminal and peritubular membranes have been assumed, because these have not yet been measured in vivo. The transepithelial P.D. declines along the length of the collecting duct, from cortex to papillary tip.

chemical potential gradient from cell into peritubular fluid and blood. It is in this segment of the nephron that extremely low Na^+ concentrations (<1.0 mEq/liter) can be attained during Na^+ deprivation. Hence, cells of the collecting duct can transport Na^+ against a very large chemical concentration gradient. As in the distal tubule, the reabsorption of Cl^- is probably largely passive except under conditions of extreme Cl^- deprivation.

The rate of water reabsorption from collecting ducts varies with the concentration of ADH, as is the case in the distal tubule (Chap. 8). When the concentration of ADH in blood is high, the rate of water reabsorption from collecting ducts is high, and vice versa.

Renal Regulation of Na+ Balance

The handling of Na^+ by the kidneys of a normal adult human is depicted in Figure 7-7, in which the single nephron represents the total function of both kidneys. With a glomerular filtration rate of 180 liters per day (see Table 1-1) and a plasma Na^+ concentration of 140 mEq/liter, the filtered load of Na^+ is

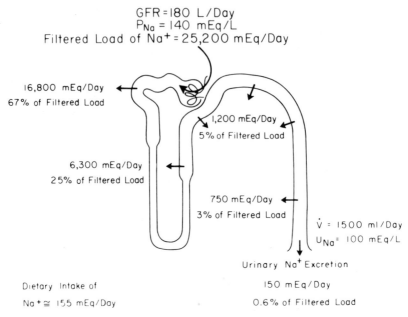

GFR = 180 L/Day
P_{Na} = 140 mEq/L
Filtered Load of Na^+ = 25,200 mEq/Day

16,800 mEq/Day
67% of Filtered Load

1,200 mEq/Day
5% of Filtered Load

6,300 mEq/Day
25% of Filtered Load

750 mEq/Day
3% of Filtered Load

$\dot{V}$ = 1500 ml/Day
U_{Na} = 100 mEq/L

Urinary Na^+ Excretion

Dietary Intake of
$Na^+ \cong$ 155 mEq/Day

150 mEq/Day
0.6% of Filtered Load

Figure 7-7

Daily renal turnover of Na^+ in a normal adult human. The diagram of the nephron represents the composite of the roughly 2 million nephrons of both kidneys. In the steady (equilibrium) state, the organism is by definition in "balance." For Na^+ this means that the daily output of Na^+ equals the daily intake. Obviously, Na^+ is excreted mainly by the kidneys; the difference between the rate of urinary excretion of Na^+ and the daily intake is made up by extrarenal routes, such as the sweat glands and the salivary glands and other gastrointestinal secretions. Under normal circumstances, the extrarenal losses of Na^+ are negligible.

180 · 140, or 25,200 mEq per day. (Strictly speaking, this value should be lowered by the Donnan factor of about 0.95; but since the value should also be raised by correcting for plasma water, the two corrections cancel one another and may be ignored. See Chap. 4.) Of the 25,200 mEq filtered, roughly 67%, or 16,800 mEq per day, is reabsorbed in the proximal tubules. Normal urine flow is about 1 ml per min; since there are 1,440 min in 24 hr, normal urine flow is about 1,500 ml per day. At a normal urinary Na^+ concentration of about 100 mEq/liter, the daily urinary excretion of Na^+ is about 150 mEq, or 0.6% of the filtered load. Hence, nearly 33% of the filtered load of Na^+ is reabsorbed beyond the proximal tubules. This is apportioned as follows: about 25% or 6,300 mEq per day in the loops of Henle; about 5% or 1,200 mEq per day in the distal tubules; and about 3% or 750 mEq per day in the collecting ducts.

Normally, then, about 99.4% of the filtered Na^+ is reabsorbed

(Table 1-1). It is obvious that, given a normal dietary intake of Na$^+$ of about 155 mEq per day, any change in the GFR or in the rate of tubular Na$^+$ reabsorption could seriously threaten the body Na$^+$ balance and hence the maintenance of the body fluid compartments (Chap. 2). Or, a change in the dietary intake of Na$^+$ would pose a similar threat unless the GFR or tubular reabsorptive rate were quickly adjusted. The fact that the plasma Na$^+$ concentration is normally carefully maintained in the narrow range of 136 to 146 mEq/liter shows that physiological adjustments must quickly come into play when Na$^+$ balance is challenged. These adjustments are discussed next.

Challenges to
Na⁺ Balance

Spontaneous Changes in GFR. Given a stable plasma concentration of Na$^+$, changes in GFR markedly alter the filtered load of Na$^+$. Hence, unless such changes were quickly accompanied by physiological adjustments, a decrease in GFR would lead to a surfeit of body Na$^+$, and an increase in GFR might lead to fatal Na$^+$ depletion. For example, if, in the case depicted in Figure 7-7, GFR *were* to increase by 25%, the filtered load of Na$^+$ would increase to 225 · 140, or 31,500 mEq per day. If the absolute amount of Na$^+$ reabsorbed *were* to remain at 25,050 mEq per day, the daily excretion of Na$^+$ would rise to 6,450 mEq, an intolerably high value. In fact, this does not happen because two physiological compensations set in: glomerulotubular balance (G-T balance) and autoregulation of GFR.

Glomerulotubular Balance. It was pointed out in Chapter 4 that when used in the context of Na$^+$ balance, G-T balance has a different connotation from the one that is derived from the glucose titration curve. In the present context, G-T balance refers to the fact that under steady-state conditions a constant fraction of the filtered Na$^+$ is reabsorbed in the proximal tubules despite variations in GFR. Normally, this fraction is about 0.67, or 67% (Fig. 7-7). If, in the hypothetical example described above, GFR had increased by 25%, G-T balance would have adjusted Na$^+$ reabsorption in the proximal tubules to 31,500 · 0.67, or about 21,100 mEq per day; if reabsorption in more distal segments were to stay the same, Na$^+$ excretion would have decreased from 6,450 to 2,150 mEq per day. Although this is an important compensation, it clearly would not suffice to prevent Na$^+$ depletion, since a Na$^+$ excretion rate of 2,000 mEq per day would still exceed the normal daily Na$^+$ intake by an order of magnitude. Actually, there are adjustments of Na^+ reabsorption, similar to G-T balance in the proximal tubules, in more distal segments as well. Furthermore, sustained large increases in GFR are usually prevented by the additional physiological adjustment of auto-regulation of GFR.

Despite a great deal of investigation, the mechanism for G-T balance remains unknown. It might involve changes in tubular flow velocity, changes in the geometry of the tubules and hence in the reabsorptive surface area, changes in the Starling forces, which govern fluid exchange across capillary walls (see Fig. 2-5), especially the oncotic and hydrostatic pressures within peri-tubular capillaries, and/or some humoral substance.

Autoregulation of GFR. This phenomenon, which is illustrated in Figure 6-4, involves the relative constancy of the total filtration rate (GFR), and possibly the glomerular filtration rate of individual nephrons (gfr) as well (Chap. 6). Whenever there is a tendency for the GFR to increase, whether it be through increased renal arterial perfusion pressure (Fig. 6-4) or through some other means, a negative feedback mechanism is activated, which tends to return the GFR to the normal level. This feedback may involve the juxtaglomerular apparatus (JGA). Whatever the mechanism, it seems likely that autoregulation is a major means whereby serious Na^+ wastage is prevented.

Thus, the threat to Na^+ balance that would be occasioned by spontaneous changes in GFR is ordinarily combatted by relative constancy of the so-called proximal fractional reabsorption (G-T balance), possibly by a similar balance in more distal segments, and by a feedback mechanism that tends quickly to return the GFR toward the normal level (autoregulation).

Changes in Na^+ Intake. Abrupt changes in the acquisition of Na^+ pose a second major threat to Na^+ balance. For example, unless a sharp decrease in Na^+ intake were accompanied by decreased excretion, Na^+, and hence fluid volume depletion, would quickly ensue. Conversely, a sudden large increase in Na^+ intake might quickly lead to an increase in total body Na^+ followed by expansion of the fluid compartments and heart failure — unless there were a rapid increase in the urinary excretion of Na^+. Physiological adjustments do in fact set in, and we shall now consider them from the point of view of compensating for increases in Na^+ intake.

Increase in GFR (First Factor). An increase in Na^+ intake is accompanied by an increase in GFR. This occurs partly because expansion of the extracellular fluid volume, which is brought about by increased Na^+ (see Fig. 2-4), is accompanied by decreased plasma oncotic pressure and often by increased arterial blood pressure, and partly for as yet unknown reasons. The increased GFR raises the filtered load of Na^+ and, other things being equal, the urinary excretion of Na^+. The argument may seem self-contradictory, since we have just reviewed physiological compensations that minimize Na^+ excretion when GFR is increased. The solution to this apparent paradox lies in the distinction between a spontaneous (primary) and a compensatory (secondary) increase in GFR. When the latter occurs, as in response to augmented Na^+ intake, it is usually not accompanied by G-T balance or by autoregulation. That is, whatever the mechanisms are that bring about G-T balance and autoregulation, these mechanisms appear to be minimized or abolished by a high intake of Na^+.

Decreased Aldosterone (Second Factor). The production of aldosterone is decreased as Na^+ intake is increased. A low blood concentration of aldosterone leads to decreased tubular reabsorption of Na^+. This effect may involve mainly the thick ascending limbs of Henle, distal tubules, and collecting ducts.

Other Factors. For many years it was thought that the first two factors cited above could wholly account for the increased urinary excretion of Na^+ that follows increased Na^+ intake. In 1961, however, H. E. de Wardener and his associates showed conclusively that under some experimental conditions these two factors did not suffice and that it was therefore necessary to invoke another factor or factors. An experiment of the type that led to this conclusion is shown in Figure 7-8. This experiment was carried out on a dog that was given high doses of aldosterone in order to rule out alterations in the blood concentration of this hormone as a cause of the observed changes. During the control periods, the dog filtered about 5 mEq of Na^+ per minute. He excreted about 0.04 mEq per minute, i.e., he reabsorbed about 99.2% of the filtered Na^+. He was then given an intravenous infusion of 0.9% NaCl, which has a Na^+ concentration of about 140 mEq/liter and therefore does not change the plasma concentration of Na^+. Ninety minutes later the urinary excretion of Na^+ had risen to 0.48 mEq per minute; however, at this point, the increment in the filtered load of Na^+ (consequent upon an increase in GFR) could more than account for the increment in Na^+ excretion. The GFR was then reduced by tightening a clamp around the aorta, just above the renal arteries. This maneuver greatly reduced the filtered load of Na^+ to about 2.9 mEq per minute. Nevertheless, with the continuance of the saline infusion, increased Na^+ excretion remained at about 0.25 mEq per minute.

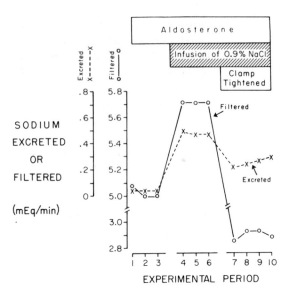

Figure 7-8

An experiment in a dog, showing conclusively that an increase in glomerular filtration rate (and hence in the filtered load of Na^+), and a decrease in aldosterone, cannot fully. account for the increased Na^+ excretion that follows an infusion of NaCl. This fact was first demonstrated conclusively by de Wardener and his associates in 1961; the experiment depicted here was taken from Levinsky, N. G. *Ann. N.Y. Acad. Sci.* 139:295, 1966. In addition to the aldosterone, the dog also received large amounts of antidiuretic hormone (ADH), thereby also ruling out alterations in the concentration of this hormone as a cause of the observed changes.

The conclusion from this type of experiment is that the increased Na^+ excretion that follows saline loading cannot be fully accounted for by increased GFR (the first factor) and therefore must be due to decreased tubular reabsorption. Since high doses of aldosterone were given throughout this experiment, the decreased reabsorption could not be ascribed to a decreased blood concentration of aldosterone (the second factor), and was therefore ascribed to a third factor or factors. This conclusion has been confirmed by micropuncture techniques. It was found by analysis of tubular fluid to plasma (TF/P) inulin (Chap. 3) that acute saline loading decreased the proportion of the filtered Na^+ (and often the absolute amount of Na^+) that is reabsorbed in proximal tubules, from the normal of about 67% to about 40%. The additional factor or factors also inhibit the reabsorption of Na^+ beyond the proximal tubules.

The additional factors have not been conclusively identified.

There are a number of possibilities, and the following list is not exhaustive. (1) *Hormone.* Investigators have long searched for a humoral substance, and some (but not others) believe that they have isolated the so-called natriuretic hormone. For a while this elusive substance was called "Third Factor"; but since the very existence of the hormone remains in doubt, and since more than a single additional factor may be involved, the term should be discarded. (2) *Change in gfr.* When animals are put on a high Na^+ intake, there is an increase in the gfr of superficial cortical nephrons (see Table 6-1). These nephrons have shorter proximal tubules than juxtamedullary nephrons, and they may thus have a lesser capacity for reabsorbing Na^+ than do the deeper ones. It has been suggested that the increase in superficial gfr may augment Na^+ excretion by placing the increased filtered load of Na^+ principally into nephrons having a lesser Na^+ reabsorbing capacity. (3) *Starling forces.* A possible scheme of how these forces might change following increased Na^+ intake is diagrammed in Figure 7-9. It is proposed that an increased Na^+ intake increases the hydrostatic pressure and decreases the plasma oncotic pressure within the peritubular capillaries. These changes

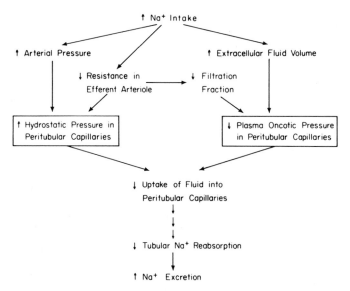

Figure 7-9
Proposed scheme whereby increased Na^+ intake might lead to increased Na^+ excretion through changes in Starling forces across peritubular capillaries. Slightly modified from Earley, L. E., and Daugharty, T. M. *New Eng. J. Med.* 281:72, 1969.

might come about directly as a result of increased systemic arterial pressure and expansion of the extracellular fluid volume, and possibly indirectly through a postulated decrease in vascular resistance at the efferent arterioles. Such decreased resistance would permit greater transmission of the systemic arterial pressure into the peritubular capillaries; it would also decrease the filtration fraction, thereby leaving more plasma in postglomerular vessels and diluting the proteins in postglomerular blood. As a result of the changes in the two major Starling forces, the fluid uptake into peritubular capillaries would be decreased. Just how such decreased uptake diminishes net Na^+ reabsorption is uncertain. In the context of the scheme depicted in Figure 7-4, it would presumably involve changes in the intercellular spaces, such as their geometry, diffusion distances or permeabilities for Na^+, or Na^+ concentration gradients. Although a number of steps depicted in Figure 7-9 are hypothetical, there is much experimental evidence that changes in the balance of Starling forces across the walls of peritubular capillaries, especially the intracapillary hydrostatic and oncotic pressures, are associated with changes in net Na^+ reabsorption.

Summary

The amounts of H_2O, and of Na^+ with its attendant anions that are filtered every day exceed their daily intakes by more than a hundredfold (see Table 1-1). For this reason, Na^+ and H_2O balance — i.e., the balance between intake and output — depends critically on the tubular reabsorption of these substances. In most segments of the nephron, Na^+ reabsorption is active, and it is the primary process that is followed by passive reabsorption of H_2O. Possible exceptions are the thin ascending limb of Henle, in which Na^+ reabsorption may be passive, and the thick ascending limb of Henle, in which Cl^- rather than Na^+ reabsorption may be the primary event.

In proximal tubules, Na^+ is transported actively, Cl^- probably passively, and H_2O is reabsorbed passively as a consequence of the movement of NaCl. So-called isosmotic fluid reabsorption from the proximal tubules involves intercellular spaces, in which the osmotic driving force for passive H_2O reabsorption is thought to reside.

Net movement of Na^+ and H_2O in thin loops of Henle has not been fully defined. Some Na^+ may be passively secreted into thin descending limbs, and water passively reabsorbed from them. In the thin ascending limbs, Na^+ is either passively or actively reabsorbed, and probably only very little H_2O is reabsorbed.

In thick ascending limbs of Henle, either Na^+ or Cl^- is actively reabsorbed to the virtual exclusion of H_2O.

Na^+ reabsorption from distal tubules and collecting ducts is active; Cl^- reabsorption is largely passive, with a small active component when very low intratubular Cl^- concentrations are attained. Reabsorption of H_2O from distal tubules and collecting ducts is passive and varies directly with the blood concentration of the antidiuretic hormone (ADH).

Normally, about 67% of the filtered Na^+ is reabsorbed in the proximal tubules, about 25% in the loops of Henle, about 5% in the distal tubules, and nearly 3% in the collecting ducts.

There are perhaps two major threats to Na^+ balance: (a) spontaneous (primary) changes in glomerular filtration rate (GFR) and hence in the filtered load of Na^+; and (b) changes in Na^+ intake. The first threat is countered by the physiological compensations of glomerulotubular (G-T) balance and autoregulation of the GFR. Balance is usually quickly reestablished in the presence of the second threat, changes in Na^+ intake, by secondary changes in GFR (first factor), changes in the blood concentration of aldosterone (second factor), and one or more additional factors. These added factors may include, among others, humoral substances, changes in the filtration rates of single nephrons (gfr), and/or changes in the Starling forces across the walls of peritubular capillaries.

Selected References

General

Brodsky, W. A., Rehm, W. S., Dennis, W. H., and Miller, D. G. Thermodynamic analysis of the intracellular osmotic gradient hypothesis of active water transport. *Science* 121:302, 1955.

Fishman, A. P. (Ed.). Symposium on salt and water metabolism. *Circulation* 21:803, 1960. (Although in some respects slightly outdated, this excellent symposium contains valuable material. It is, in many places, enlivened by discussion that is still remembered by those who attended the meeting.)

Gottschalk, C. W. *Renal Tubular Function: Lessons From Micropuncture.* The Harvey Lectures, Series LVIII, 1962–63. Academic, New York, 1963.

Orloff, J., and Burg, M. G. Kidney. *Ann. Rev. Physiol.* 33:83, 1971.

Walser, M. Sodium Excretion. In C. Rouiller and A. F. Muller (Eds.), *The Kidney,* vol. III. Academic, New York, 1971.

Na⁺ and H₂O Transport in Various Tubular Segments

Epstein, F. H. The Role of Sodium and Potassium ATPase in Renal Sodium Reabsorption. In K. Thurau and H. Jahrmärker (Eds.), *Renal Transport and Diuretics.* Springer, New York, 1969.

Giebisch, G. Functional organization of proximal and distal tubular electrolyte transport. *Nephron* 6:260, 1969.

Giebisch, G., Boulpaep, E. L., and Whittembury, G. Electrolyte transport in kidney tubule cells. *Phil. Trans. Roy. Soc. London.* Series B. 262:175, 1971.

Giebisch, G., Klose, R. M., Malnic, G., Sullivan, W. J., and Windhager, E. E. Sodium movement across single perfused proximal tubules of rat kidneys. *J. Gen. Physiol.* 47:1175, 1964.

Giebisch, G., and Windhager, E. E. Electrolyte Transport Across Renal Tubular Membranes. In J. Orloff and R. W. Berliner (Eds.), *Handbook of Physiology.* Section 8: Renal Physiology. American Physiological Society, Washington, D.C., 1973.

Hilger, H. H., Klümper, J. D., and Ullrich, K. J. Wasserrückresorption und Ionentransport durch die Sammelrohrzellen der Säugetierniere. *Pflügers Arch. Ges. Physiol.* 267:218, 1958.

Jamison, R. L. Micropuncture study of superficial and juxtamedullary nephrons in the rat. *Amer. J. Physiol.* 218:46, 1970.

Kokko, J. P. Sodium chloride and water transport in the descending limb of Henle. *J. Clin. Invest.* 49:1838, 1970.

Marsh, D. J. Solute and water flows in thin limbs of Henle's loop in the hamster kidney. *Amer. J. Physiol.* 218:824, 1970.

Marsh, D. J., and Solomon, S. Analysis of electrolyte movement in thin Henle's loops of hamster papilla. *Amer. J. Physiol.* 208:1119, 1965.

Walker, A. M., Bott, P. A., Oliver, J., and MacDowell, M. C. The collection and analysis of fluid from single nephrons of the mammalian kidney. *Amer. J. Physiol.* 134:580, 1941.

Windhager, E. E. Electrophysiological study of renal papilla of golden hamsters. *Amer. J. Physiol.* 206:694, 1964.

Windhager, E. E., Whittembury, G., Oken, D. E., Schatzmann, H. J., and Solomon, A. K. Single proximal tubules of the *Necturus* kidney: III. Dependence of H_2O movement on NaCl concentration. *Amer. J. Physiol.* 197:313, 1959.

Fluid Transport in Epithelia

Curran, P. F. Ion transport in intestine and its coupling to other transport processes. *Fed. Proc.* 24:993, 1965.

Curran, P. F., and MacIntosh, J. R. A model system for biological water transport. *Nature* (London) 193:347, 1962.

Diamond, J. M., and Tormey, J. McD. Studies on the structural basis of water transport across epithelial membranes. *Fed. Proc.* 25:1458, 1966.

Dietschy, J. M. Recent developments in solute and water transport across the gall bladder epithelium. *Gastroenterology* 50:692, 1966.

Ganote, C. E., Grantham, J. J., Moses, H. L., Burg, M. B., and Orloff, J. Ultrastructural studies of vasopressin effect on isolated perfused renal collecting tubules of the rabbit. *J. Cell Biol.* 36:355, 1968.

Physiology Society. Comparative aspects of transport of hypertonic, isotonic, and hypotonic solutions by epithelial membranes. A Physiology Society Symposium, chaired by B. Schmidt-Nielsen. *Fed. Proc.* 30:3, 1971.

This symposium includes the following articles: (a) Standing-gradient model of fluid transport in epithelia, by J. M. Diamond; (b) Mode of water transport in mammalian renal collecting tubules, by J. J. Grantham; (c) Experimental modification of lateral and basilar plasma membranes and extracellular compartments in the flounder nephron, by B. F. Trump and R. E. Bulger; (d) Local osmotic gradients in the rectal pads of an insect, by B. J. Wall; and (e) The structural basis of fluid secretion, by J. L. Ochsman and M. J. Berridge.

Tisher, C. C., Bulger, R. E., and Valtin, H. Morphology of renal medulla in water diuresis and vasopressin-induced antidiuresis. *Amer. J. Physiol.* 220:87, 1971.

Ullrich, K. J., Rumrich, G., and Fuchs, G. Wasserpermeabilität und transtubulärer Wasserfluss corticaler Nephronabschnitte bei verschiedenen Diuresezuständen. *Pflügers Arch. Ges. Physiol.* 280:99, 1964.

Electrophysiology Malnic, G., Klose, R. M., and Giebisch, G. Microperfusion study of distal tubular potassium and sodium transfer in rat kidney. *Amer. J. Physiol.* 211:548, 1966.

Ussing, H., and Zerahn, K. Active transport of sodium as the source of electric current in the short-circuited frog skin. *Acta Physiol. Scand.* 23:110, 1951.

Windhager, E. E., and Giebisch, G. Electrophysiology of the nephron. *Physiol. Rev.* 45:214, 1965.

Wright, F. S. Increasing magnitude of electrical potential along the renal distal tubule. *Amer. J. Physiol.* 220:624, 1971.

Na⁺ Balance Blythe, W. B., D'Avila, D., Gitelman, H. J., and Welt, L. G. Further evidence for a humoral natriuretic factor. *Circ. Res.* 28(Suppl. 2): II-21, 1971.

Brown, P. R., Kontsaimanis, K. G., and de Wardener, H. E. Effect of urinary extracts from salt-loaded man on urinary sodium excretion by the rat. *Kidney Int.* 2:1, 1972.

Cort, J. H., Dousa, T., Pliska, V., Lichardus, B., Safarova, J., Vranesic, M., and Rudinger, J. Saluretic activity of blood during carotid occlusion in the cat. *Amer. J. Physiol.* 215:921, 1968.

de Wardener, H. E. Control of sodium reabsorption. *Brit. Med. J.* 3:611;676, 1969.

Kramer, K., Boylan, J. W., and Keck, W. Regulation of total body sodium in the mammalian organism. *Nephron* 6:379, 1969.

Mills, I. H. Renal regulation of sodium excretion. *Ann. Rev. Med.* 21:75, 1970.

Schrier, R. W., and de Wardener, H. E. Tubular reabsorption of sodium ion. *New Eng. J. Med.* 285:1231;1292, 1971.

Sealey, J. E., Kirshman, J. D., and Laragh, J. H. Natriuretic activity in plasma and urine of salt-loaded man and sheep. *J. Clin. Invest.* 48:2210, 1969.

Wright, F. S., Brenner, B. M., Bennett, C. M., Keimowitz, R. I., Berliner, R. W., Schrier, R. W., Verroust, P. J., de Wardener, H. E., and Holzgreve, H. Failure to demonstrate a hormonal inhibitor of proximal sodium reabsorption. *J. Clin. Invest.* 48:1107, 1969.

Aldosterone Davis, J. O. The Renin-Angiotensin System in the Control of
and Renin Aldosterone Secretion. In J. W. Fisher (Ed.), *Kidney Hormones.* Academic, New York, 1971.

Edelman, I. S., and Fimognari, G. M. On the biochemical mechanism of action of aldosterone. *Recent Progr. Hormone Res.* 24:1, 1968.

Finn, A. L., and Welt, L. G. Effect of aldosterone administration on electrolyte excretion and GFR in the rat. *Amer. J. Physiol.* 204:243, 1963.

Hierholzer, K., and Stolte, H. The proximal and distal tubular action of adrenal steroids on Na reabsorption. *Nephron* 6:188, 1969.

Mulrow, P. J. The adrenal cortex. *Ann. Rev. Physiol.* 34:409, 1972.

Sharp, G. W. G., and Leaf, A. Aldosterone. In J. Orloff and R. W. Berliner (Eds.), *Handbook of Physiology.* Section 8: Renal Physiology. American Physiological Society, Washington, D.C., 1973.

Symposium on aldosterone and active sodium transport across epithelia. *J. Steroid Biochem.* 3:105, 1972.

Peritubular Control of Fluid Reabsorption

Brenner, B. M., and Galla, J. H. Influence of postglomerular hematocrit and protein concentration on rat nephron fluid transfer. *Amer. J. Physiol.* 220:148, 1971.

Brenner, B. M., and Troy, J. L. Postglomerular vascular protein concentration: Evidence for a causal role in governing fluid reabsorption and glomerulotubular balance by the renal proximal tubule. *J. Clin. Invest.* 50:336, 1971.

de Wardener, H. E., Mills, I. H., Clapham, W. F., and Hayter, C. J. Studies on the efferent mechanism of the sodium diuresis which follows the administration of intravenous saline in the dog. *Clin. Sci.* 21:249, 1961.

Earley, L. E. Influence of hemodynamic factors on sodium reabsorption. *Ann. N.Y. Acad. Sci.* 139:312, 1966.

Earley, L. E., and Schrier, R. W. Intrarenal Control of Sodium Excretion by Hemodynamic and Physical Factors. In J. Orloff and R. W. Berliner (Eds.), *Handbook of Physiology.* Section 8: Renal Physiology. American Physiological Society, Washington, D.C., 1973.

Falchuk, K. H., Brenner, B. M., Tadokoro, M., and Berliner, R. W. Oncotic and hydrostatic pressures in peritubular capillaries and fluid reabsorption by proximal tubule. *Amer. J. Physiol.* 220:1427, 1971.

Howards, S. S., Davis, B. B., Knox, F. G., Wright, F. S., and Berliner, R. W. Depression of fractional sodium reabsorption by the proximal tubule of the dog without sodium diuresis. *J. Clin. Invest.* 47:1561, 1968.

Levy, M., and Levinsky, N. G. Proximal reabsorption and intrarenal pressure during colloid infusions in the dog. *Amer. J. Physiol.* 220:415, 1971.

Share, L., and Claybaugh, J. R. Regulation of body fluids. *Ann. Rev. Physiol.* 34:235, 1972.

Windhager, E. E., Lewy, J. E., and Spitzer, A. Intrarenal control of proximal tubular reabsorption of sodium and water. *Nephron* 6:247, 1969.

Glomerulotubular Balance

Arrizurieta-Muchnik, E. E., Lassiter, W. E., Lipham, E. M., and Gottschalk, C. W. Micropuncture study of glomerulotubular balance in the rat kidney. *Nephron* 6:418, 1969.

Brenner, B. M., Bennett, C. M., and Berliner, R. W. The relationship between glomerular filtration rate and sodium reabsorption by the proximal tubule of the rat nephron. *J. Clin. Invest.* 47:1358, 1968.

Burg, M. B., and Orloff, J. Control of fluid absorption in the renal proximal tubule. *J. Clin. Invest.* 47:2016, 1968.

Gertz, K. H. Glomerular Tubular Balance. In J. Orloff and R. W. Berliner (Eds.), *Handbook of Physiology.* Section 8: Renal Physiology. American Physiological Society, Washington, D.C., 1973.

Divalent Cations

Epstein, F. H. Calcium and the kidney. *Amer. J. Med.* 45:700, 1968.

Walser, M. Divalent Cations: Physicochemical State in Glomerular Filtrate and Urine, and Renal Excretion. In J. Orloff and R. W. Berliner (Eds.), *Handbook of Physiology.* Section 8: Renal Physiology. American Physiological Society, Washington, D.C., 1973.

8 : Concentration and Dilution of Urine: H_2O Balance

Even though water reabsorption is a passive event that follows the reabsorption of Na^+, water balance can be regulated independently of Na^+ balance. This is accomplished through changes in the blood concentration of the antidiuretic hormone (ADH or vasopressin), which adjusts the amount of water that is reabsorbed from the distal tubules and collecting ducts. When the concentration of ADH is high, so is the water permeability of these nephron segments. Consequently, much water is reabsorbed and hyperosmotic urine is formed (up to about 1,200 mOsm/kg H_2O in man). Conversely, a low concentration of ADH reduces the water permeability of distal tubules and collecting ducts. This results in little water reabsorption from these segments and the formation of hyposmotic urine (down to about 50 mOsm/kg H_2O in man).

The Countercurrent Mechanism As we have seen, in all nephron segments except perhaps the thin limbs of the loops of Henle, the transport of Na^+ (or possibly Cl^- in the thick ascending limbs of Henle) is active, while water reabsorption is passive. Given these prerequisites, it is conceptually easy to form hyposmotic urine: the kidneys actively reabsorb Na^+ (and its anions) from an isosmotic glomerular filtrate while much of the water is retained within the tubules. It proved more difficult, however, to conceive a system that will produce hyperosmotic urine through the passive reabsorption of water, as this requires the buildup of large osmotic gradients in the tissues surrounding the tubules. The problem of hyperosmotic urine formation through passive water reabsorption puzzled renal physiologists for many years until W. Kuhn and K. Ryffel proposed the countercurrent mechanism. The principle of this mechanism in a normal human being concentrating his urine to 1,200 mOsm/kg H_2O is illustrated in Figure 8-1.

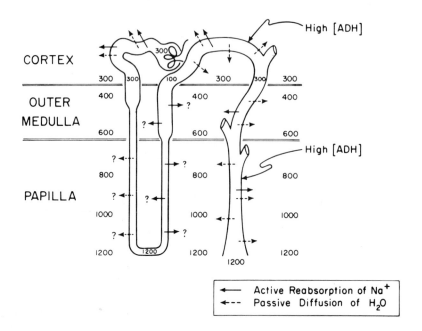

Figure 8-1

Operation of the countercurrent mechanism in normal man during antidiuresis. The numbers refer to the osmolality (mOsm/kg H_2O) of either intratubular or interstitial fluid. Solid arrows denote active reabsorption of Na^+ (its accompanying anions, mainly Cl^-, being reabsorbed passively); arrows with a dashed line denote passive reabsorption of water. The question marks in the loops of Henle indicate that it is not yet known: (a) how much H_2O is reabsorbed from descending limbs; (b) whether solute transport out of thin ascending limbs is active or passive; and (c) whether Na^+ or Cl^- is actively reabsorbed from thick ascending limbs. The number of arrows in each nephron segment signifies semiquantitatively the amounts of solute transported relative to water. For example, in ascending limbs of Henle, solute is reabsorbed to the virtual but not complete exclusion of water, since renal membranes are not absolutely impervious to water.

Formation of
Hyperosmotic
(Concentrated)
Urine

This is thought to occur through the following sequence of events:

1. The fluid in Bowman's capsule, being an ultrafiltrate of plasma, has an osmolality of about 300 mOsm/kg H_2O.
2. About two-thirds of the glomerular filtrate is reabsorbed isosmotically in the proximal tubule (also see Figs. 7-3 and 7-7). Hence, intratubular fluid at the end of the proximal tubule still has an osmolality of 300 mOsm/kg H_2O.
3. The wall of the ascending limb of Henle is thought to be relatively impermeable to water. Therefore, in this segment Na^+ is reabsorbed to the virtual exclusion of water, a process that renders the medullary and papillary inter-

stitium hyperosmotic to plasma. This process is abetted by the loops of Henle acting as countercurrent multipliers (see below). Since isosmotic fluid entered the loops of Henle and Na^+ (with its anions) was withdrawn, intratubular fluid at the beginning of the distal tubule is hyposmotic.

4. With a high concentration of ADH in the blood, the membranes lining the distal tubules and collecting ducts are highly permeable to water. Hence, all along these tubular segments, water diffuses passively down the osmotic gradient between intratubular fluid and cortical, medullary, and papillary interstitium. The tubular fluid is thereby concentrated until osmotic equilibrium with the interstitium is reached, and this progressive concentration of intratubular fluid takes place even though some Na^+ continues to be reabsorbed from the distal tubules and collecting ducts.

This is called the countercurrent system, for at least three reasons: (a) the loops of Henle act as countercurrent multipliers; (b) the vasa recta act as countercurrent exchangers (see below); and (c) it is the countercurrent arrangement of the entire nephron that gives the urine a chance to flow through an area of hyperosmolality, thereby permitting concentration of urine through the passive reabsorption of water.

Formation of Hyposmotic (Dilute) Urine

During the formation of dilute urine, the sequence is qualitatively identical up to the beginning of the distal tubule. Now, however, the blood concentration of ADH is low or zero, so that the membranes lining the distal tubules and collecting ducts are relatively impermeable to water. Hence, less water is reabsorbed than during antidiuresis, even though an osmotic gradient between tubular lumen and interstitium persists. Na^+ continues to be reabsorbed, which further helps to dilute the urine.

Historical Hints

It is of interest that although the countercurrent hypothesis became accepted as the mechanism only around 1960, strong hints on where to search for the mechanism were extant in the literature for at least 50 years. In 1909, K. Peter pointed to the correlation between the length of thin loops of Henle in different species of mammals and the degree to which they could concentrate the urine. For example, in the kangaroo rat, which lives in the desert and can concentrate its urine to at least 5,500 mOsm/kg H_2O, some long loops of Henle reach all the way into the ureter; whereas in rodents that do not live in an arid habitat and concentrate their urine to about 2,500 mOsm /kg H_2O the long loops are not nearly so long, reaching only to the tip of the papilla. In 1925, E. H. Starling and E. B. Verney pointed out (albeit in a footnote) that there is a correspondence between the ability to make urine hyperosmotic to plasma, and the presence of medullary loops of Henle. This point was again emphasized by E. K. Marshall, Jr., in 1934, by showing that only birds and mammals could render urine hyperosmotic to plasma, and only in these animals did one find medullary loops of Henle (see Fig. 1-4).

All this evidence suggested to investigators that urine must be concentrated within the loops of Henle. Then micropuncture studies showed that tubular fluid even in late portions of the distal tubules is either hyposmotic or isosmotic, but not hyperosmotic. It therefore was clear that the fluid must become hyperosmotic in the collecting ducts.

The correct role of the loops of Henle was first suggested in 1942 by two Swiss workers, W. Kuhn and K. Ryffel, who published a paper entitled "Production of concentrated solutions from diluted ones solely by membrane effects: A model for renal function." However, their countercurrent theory was largely ignored because it seemed unnecessarily complicated compared to active reabsorption of water. Nevertheless, the Swiss group persisted, and in 1951 H. Wirz, B. Hargitay, and W. Kuhn reproposed the countercurrent theory and presented preliminary experimental evidence (discussed below) supporting their hypothesis. By 1960 the experimental evidence in its favor became so overwhelming that the hypothesis was accepted.

Countercurrent Multiplication in Loops of Henle

A schema for countercurrent multiplication is depicted in Figure 8-2. This type of process, or some modification thereof, occurs in the loops of Henle. Two apposing tubes are separated by a membrane that is impermeable to water. (For the sake of clarity, the membrane is considered absolutely impermeable in this example; actually, it is only relatively impermeable to water.) Fluid in the two tubes flows in opposite directions. At any horizontal level, Na^+ (and with it, Cl^-) can be transported out of the ascending limb to create a maximum osmotic gradient of 200 mOsm/kg H_2O. Fluid within the loops is then concentrated by the following sequence of events:

SCHEMA FOR COUNTERCURRENT MULTIPLICATION IN LOOPS OF HENLE

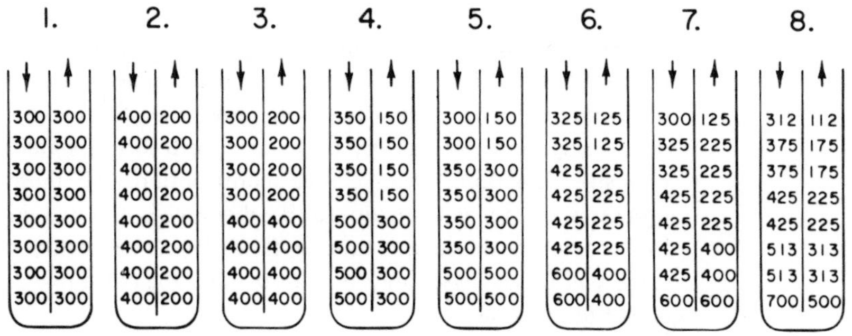

1.		2.		3.		4.		5.		6.		7.		8.	
300	300	400	200	300	200	350	150	300	150	325	125	300	125	312	112
300	300	400	200	300	200	350	150	300	150	325	125	325	225	375	175
300	300	400	200	300	200	350	150	350	300	425	225	325	225	375	175
300	300	400	200	300	200	350	150	350	300	425	225	425	225	425	225
300	300	400	200	400	400	500	300	350	300	425	225	425	225	425	225
300	300	400	200	400	400	500	300	350	300	425	225	425	400	513	313
300	300	400	200	400	400	500	300	500	500	600	400	425	400	513	313
300	300	400	200	400	400	500	300	500	500	600	400	600	600	700	500

Figure 8-2
A countercurrent multiplier system as it might exist in the loops of Henle. The membrane separating the limbs is impermeable to water, and it can transport Na^+ and Cl^- to build up an osmotic gradient of 200 mOsm/kg H_2O at any given horizontal level. This process of transporting solute without water is known as the *single effect,* which is multiplied. Adapted from Pitts, R. F. *Physiology of the Kidney and Body Fluids,* 2d ed. Year Book, Chicago, 1968.

1. The system is filled with isosmotic fluid emanating from the proximal tubule.
2. An osmotic gradient of 200 mOsm/kg H_2O is established by transport of Na^+ and Cl^- from the ascending to the descending limb of the loop of Henle. Na^+ (or Cl^-) transport is active in thick ascending limbs; it may or may not be active in thin ascending limbs.
3. More isosmotic fluid comes into the descending limb, pushing hyposmotic fluid out of the ascending limb and into the early distal tubule.
4. A gradient of 200 mOsm/kg H_2O is again established by transporting Na^+ and Cl^- out of the ascending and into the descending limb.
5. More isosmotic fluid enters the system, pushing hyposmotic fluid into the distal tubule (and so on through Steps 6, 7, and 8).

Note the following points. (1) By Step 8, the concentration at the bend of the loop is nearly 400 mOsm/kg H_2O higher than at the beginning of the descending limb, even though transport of Na^+ and Cl^- could generate a maximum gradient of only 200 mOsm/kg H_2O at any given horizontal level; that is, the so-called "single effect" of transporting solute without water gets multiplied in this kind of system. (2) The longer the countercurrent loops of Henle, the greater will be the concentration at the bend of the loop. (3) The descending and ascending limbs of Henle need not be contiguous in order for the system to operate; there may be interstitial tissue between them. (4) Fluid within the descending thin limb becomes increasingly concentrated (Fig. 8-1). This may occur partly by passive diffusion of Na^+ and Cl^- from the interstitium into the descending limbs, and partly by passive diffusion of water in the opposite direction. The relative contributions of these two processes are not yet known. (5) By themselves, the two limbs of Henle actually dilute the tubular fluid. Hyperosmolality of the urine will be achieved only if a third tube, the collecting duct, is added to the system.

Countercurrent Exchange in Vasa Recta

Only about 5% of the total renal blood flow (RBF) (see Table 6-2), and hence of the total renal plasma flow (RPF), courses through the outer medulla and papilla. Nevertheless, the amount of plasma entering the medulla exceeds the flow of tubular fluid at the beginning of the collecting ducts by a factor of about 10. For example, 5% of a normal RPF of 660 ml per minute is 33 ml per minute, while the flow of fluid at the beginning of the collecting ducts is about 3% of the glomerular filtration rate (GFR), or 3 to 4 ml per minute. Since the vasa recta are probably highly permeable to water and are also surrounded by hyperosmotic interstitium, it would seem at first glance that the countercurrent mechanism might be concentrating about 10 ml of plasma for every 1 ml of urine. In fact, this seemingly inefficient system for concentrating urine is prevented by the countercurrent flow of blood in the vasa recta.

The countercurrent exchange system in the vasa recta is illustrated in Figure 8-3. This system prevents undue concentration of plasma as it leaves the kidney, in the following manner:

1. Blood enters the vasa recta at a concentration of about 300 mOsm/kg H_2O.
2. As this blood flows through medullary and papillary interstitium of increasing osmolality, solute diffuses passively down its concentration gradient into the descending limb of vasa recta, and water passively diffuses out of this limb in response to the osmotic gradient. This process results in increasing osmolality within the vasa recta as the bend is approached.
3. As the blood rises in the ascending limb of the vasa recta, it encounters less and less concentrated medullary inter-

COUNTERCURRENT EXCHANGE IN VASA RECTA

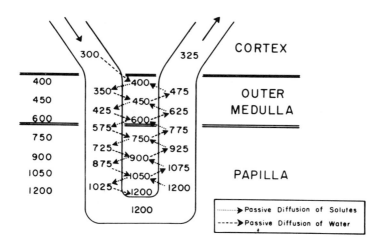

Figure 8-3

The countercurrent exchange system in the vasa recta. Arrows with dotted lines denote passive transport of solutes; arrows with dashed lines denote passive movement of water. The numbers refer to osmolalities (mOsm/kg H$_2$O) in the blood or interstitial fluid. Adapted from Berliner, R. W., Levinsky, N. G., Davidson, D. G., and Eden, M. *Amer. J. Med.* 24:730, 1958.

stitium. Hence solutes passively diffuse into the interstitium and water diffuses back into the vasa recta.

Note that as a result of this passive countercurrent exchange, blood leaves the kidneys not at 1,200 mOsm/kg H$_2$O (as it would in a straight flow system) but at about 325 mOsm/kg H$_2$O. Thus, concentration of blood, and hence depletion of medullary and papillary solutes by the blood flow, are greatly minimized although not wholly prevented.

It might be asked why, if blood flow is such a threat to the renal concentrating mechanism, must blood course through the medulla and papilla at all. There are at least two reasons: (a) there must be nutrient blood flow to the medullary and papillary tissues; and (b) the water that is reabsorbed from the collecting ducts must be removed from the inner regions of the kidney by the vasa recta, lest these regions swell uncontrollably.

Experimental Evidence for the Countercurrent System

Table 8-1 lists some conditions that must be met if the countercurrent hypothesis is correct, and the experimental proof that the conditions are met.

Table 8-1
Experimental proof for the countercurrent mechanism.

Condition	Proof
1. Osmolalities of the tubular fluid along the nephron are as follows:	
During formation of hyperosmotic urine:	
Isosmotic in Bowman's space	Micropuncture (Fig. 8-1)
Isosmotic at end of proximal tubule	Micropuncture (Fig. 8-1)
Hyperosmotic at bend of loop of Henle	Micropuncture (Fig. 8-1)
Hyposmotic at beginning of distal tubule	Micropuncture (Fig. 8-1)
Isosmotic at end of distal tubule	Micropuncture (Fig. 8-1)
Hyperosmotic at end of collecting duct	Micropuncture (Fig. 8-1)
During formation of hyposmotic urine:	
Same as above through beginning of distal tubule	Micropuncture
Hyposmotic at end of distal tubule	Micropuncture
Hyposmotic at end of collecting duct	Micropuncture
2. During antidiuresis, osmolalities at any given level perpendicular to the cortico-papillary axis should be about equal.	Micropuncture, and cryoscopy of renal tissue slices. At any given horizontal level, the osmolality is about the same in the loops of Henle, collecting ducts, interstitium, and vasa recta. During water diuresis (formation of hyposmotic urine), fluid in distal tubules and collecting ducts is hyposmotic to plasma and to fluid in the other structures.
3. The osmolality of the interstitium must increase as the renal papilla is approached; i.e., there must be a so-called cortico-papillary osmotic gradient.	Cryoscopy of renal tissue slices, and chemical analysis of tissue homogenates. The cryoscopic data constituted the first experimental support for the hypothesis; they were published by Wirz, Hargitay, and Kuhn in 1951.
4. If the major change in the system between forming hyperosmotic rather than hyposmotic urine is the water permeability of the distal tubules and collecting ducts, the medullary and papillary interstitium should be hyperosmotic even during water diuresis.	Micropuncture, cryoscopy of renal tissue slices, and chemical analysis of tissue homogenates. The condition is met, but the degree of interstitial hyperosmolality is much less in water diuresis than in antidiuresis. For example, in water diuresis the papillary interstitium has an osmolality of 500 to 600 mOsm/kg H_2O. Not all the reasons for the difference have been identified; they include decreased reabsorption of urea into the medullary and papillary interstitium (see below), and probably depletion of interstitial solutes (so-called "washout") by increased blood flow through the medulla and papilla.

Role of Urea in the Counter-current System

The principles of the countercurrent mechanism can be understood by considering the transport merely of Na^+, Cl^-, and water, as we have done. Urea, however, plays an additional and important role.

In the text of Chapter 4 and in Figure 4-4, we presented the fact that more urea is reabsorbed from the collecting ducts at low urine flows, when hyperosmotic urine is formed, than at high flows. Urea deposition into the medullary and papillary interstitium is also aided by the process of medullary recycling of urea (Fig. 4-5), which delivers more urea to the collecting ducts than would be the case if recycling did not occur. Finally, urea reabsorption from collecting ducts is abetted at low urine flows (antidiuresis) by a differential effect of ADH on the urea and water permeabilities of the distal tubules and collecting ducts (Fig. 8-4). ADH increases the *water* permeability of the distal tubule and the *entire* collecting duct; however, it increases the *urea* permeability only of that portion of the collecting duct that passes through the medulla and papilla, the so-called late or medullary collecting duct. Even in the presence of ADH, the distal tubule and early (or cortical) collecting duct have a very low permeability for urea. Consequently, as water is withdrawn from the distal tubules and early collecting ducts during the formation of hyperosmotic urine, the urea, unable to diffuse out of the lumen as readily as water, is progressively concentrated. When the fluid reaches the late collecting ducts, the concentrated urea diffuses into the medullary and papillary interstitium until

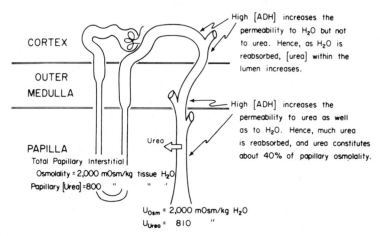

Figure 8-4
Some of the major mechanisms whereby urea increases the osmolality of the papillary interstitium, and hence aids the conservation of water. Brackets denote concentrations. The data were obtained in rats, and have been adapted from Valtin, H. *J. Clin. Invest.* 45:337, 1966.

its concentration at any given level in the interstitium is equal to its concentration at the same level in the collecting ducts. As a result of these processes that promote its reabsorption, urea constitutes about 40% of the total medullary and papillary solute concentration during antidiuresis, whereas it contributes less than 10% to the interstitial osmolality during water diuresis.

Urea is the major end product of protein metabolism in mammals, and it is excreted almost solely by the kidneys. Usually when a solute is excreted in the urine, it obligates the simultaneous excretion of water. This is so because the solute contributes to the osmolality of the tubular fluid and thereby decreases the osmotic gradient (which governs the passive reabsorption of water) between tubular lumen and interstitium. The classic example is osmotic diuresis, as induced by mannitol. Mannitol is a small solute that, for practical purposes, is not reabsorbed by the tubules. When mannitol is given intravenously, and thence filtered, it raises the osmolality of tubular fluid and decreases the reabsorption of water, so that a diuresis ensues. In the case of urea, however, that portion of the osmolality within late collecting ducts that is due to urea is balanced by an equal concentration of urea in the interstitium surrounding the collecting ducts (Fig. 8-4). Hence, urea can be excreted in the urine without obligating the simultaneous excretion of large amounts of water. This "economy of water" has been recognized for years as a unique feature of the major solute end product of mammalian protein metabolism; it is of obvious advantage for organisms that must avidly conserve water in order to survive.

Unresolved Questions

Although it is generally agreed that urine is concentrated by a combination of countercurrent multiplication and countercurrent exchange, it must be stressed that the mammalian system does not necessarily operate precisely as it has been described in this chapter. Major unsolved questions include: (a) the means whereby the osmolality of fluid within the descending limb of Henle rises (Fig. 8-1), whether primarily by solute entry or by water abstraction, or through both; (b) whether the reabsorption of Na^+ (Cl^-) from the thin ascending limb is active or passive; and (c) whether urea plays a role in addition to that which has been outlined above. These unsolved questions are considered in several of the references that have been listed at the end of this chapter.

Antidiuresis and Water Diuresis

The classic experiments of E. B. Verney in the early 1940s elucidated some of the major mechanisms that regulate the secretion of ADH from the posterior pituitary. These experiments are diagrammed in Figure 8-5a. Verney worked with trained, unanesthetized dogs in which he had exteriorized loops of both common carotid arteries, prior to carrying out the experiments. He observed that within 60 to 90 minutes after receiving a large oral load of tap water, these dogs excreted large amounts of hyposmotic urine. This water diuresis could be abruptly interrupted by infusing a bolus of hyperosmotic solution into the exteriorized carotid loop, but not if the posterior pituitary gland had been removed. If posterior pituitary extract was given to an hypophysectomized animal, the water diuresis was also interrupted.

On the basis of these results, Verney proposed the scheme outlined in Figure 8-5b. When an individual is deprived of water, the continued obligatory excretion of water renders his plasma hyperosmotic. This change stimulates osmoreceptors that

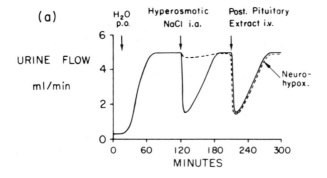

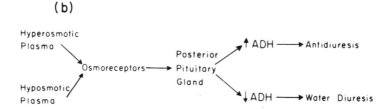

Figure 8-5
(a) Summary of some of the important results obtained on unanesthetized dogs by E. B. Verney. *Proc. Roy. Soc. London,* Series B. 135:25, 1947. Solid line graph represents results on a dog prior to removal of the neurohypophysis; the dashed line represents results on the same dog after neurohypophysectomy. p.o. = per os (by mouth); i.a. = intra-arterially (into the exteriorized loop of the common carotid artery); i.v. = intravenously.
(b) Chain of events whereby changes in plasma osmolality regulate antidiuretic hormone (ADH) secretion and hence urine flow. Although other factors — e.g., emotion, alcohol, extracellular fluid volume — can also affect ADH secretion, the osmoreceptor system is probably the major mechanism for regulating water balance.

generate afferent signals calling for the secretion of an antidiuretic substance, which has since been identified as ADH. The
resulting high concentration of ADH in the blood then leads to
antidiuresis, now known to be mediated mainly through increased
water permeability of the distal tubules and collecting ducts.

Conversely, when the individual drinks a large amount of
dilute fluid, his plasma becomes hyposmotic. This, Verney
proposed, sets off the opposite chain of events, leading to a
decreased concentration of ADH in the blood, decreased water
permeability of the distal tubules and collecting ducts, and water
diuresis.

Since prior removal of the pars nervosa abolished the response
to hyperosmotic solutions, Verney surmised that the antidiuretic
substance came from the posterior pituitary gland. This suspicion
was supported by the antidiuretic response to posterior pituitary
extract. The osmoreceptors have never been identified anatom-
ically; they presumably lie within the distribution of the internal
carotid artery.

As is shown in Figure 8-5a, modulations in ADH secretion, and
hence in urine flow, occur very rapidly, within a few minutes.
Thus, both the pituitary and the renal components of this system
comprise a fairly sensitive and precise mechanism for maintaining
water balance.

Free Water

Free water refers to water that is free of solutes. In the kidney,
free water is produced or "generated" in the ascending limbs of
Henle where relatively more Na^+ and Cl^- than water are
reabsorbed. Whether or not free water is excreted in the urine
depends on ADH and the water permeability of the distal tubules
and collecting ducts. If the concentration of ADH in blood is low,
much of the free water that was generated in the ascending limbs
will not be reabsorbed, and hyposmotic urine will be excreted.
Relative to the isosmotic plasma that was filtered, more water
than solute will have been excreted, and in this sense the net
result will be that free water has been removed or cleared from
the plasma. When the concentration of ADH is high, all the
generated free water, and more, will be reabsorbed and hyperosmotic urine will be excreted. The excretion of hyperosmotic
urine reflects a net process in which relatively more solute than
water was removed from isosmotic plasma. In this sense, no free
water will have been removed or cleared from the plasma; in fact,
a negative quantity of free water will have been cleared.

Free-Water Clearance. The view that the excretion of

hyposmotic or hyperosmotic urine represents the clearance of a positive and negative quantity of free water, respectively, from isosmotic plasma, led to the expression "free-water clearance" (C_{H_2O}). This is unfortunate, for unlike all other renal clearances, C_{H_2O} is *not* equal to $U_{H_2O} \cdot \dot{V}/P_{H_2O}$. However, the term is so well established in renal physiology that any attempt to change it is likely to cause more confusion than enlightenment. Hence, the term will be used in this book, but with the admonition that *it is not a classic renal clearance.*

Free-water clearance may be defined as the amount of distilled water that must be subtracted from or added to the urine in order to render that urine isosmotic with plasma. The formula for calculating this amount of distilled water is as follows:

$$C_{H_2O} = \dot{V} - C_{Osm} \tag{8-1}$$

where C_{Osm} = the osmolal clearance, or $U_{Osm} \cdot \dot{V}/P_{Osm}$.
When a hyposmotic urine of 100 mOsm/kg H_2O is formed, and the urine flow is 10 ml per minute

$$C_{H_2O} = \frac{10 \text{ ml}}{\text{min}} - \left(\frac{100 \text{ mOsm}}{1000 \text{ ml}} \cdot \frac{10 \text{ ml}}{\text{min}} \cdot \frac{1000 \text{ ml}}{300 \text{ mOsm}} \right)$$

$$C_{H_2O} = 6.7 \text{ ml/min}$$

When a hyperosmotic urine of 1,000 mOsm/kg H_2O is formed, and the urine flow is 0.5 ml per minute

$$C_{H_2O} = \frac{0.5 \text{ ml}}{\text{min}} - \left(\frac{1000 \text{ mOsm}}{1000 \text{ ml}} \cdot \frac{0.5 \text{ ml}}{\text{min}} \cdot \frac{1000 \text{ ml}}{300 \text{ mOsm}} \right)$$

$$C_{H_2O} = - 1.2 \text{ ml/min}$$

That is, when hyposmotic urine is formed, the free-water clearance has a positive value, and when hyperosmotic urine is formed, this clearance has a negative value. Obviously, when the urine is isosmotic with plasma, C_{H_2O} will be zero.

In order to circumvent the awkward expression *negative free-water clearance,* the term $T^c_{H_2O}$ was coined. This refers to the net transport of free water in a reabsorptive direction when hyperosmotic urine is formed; the superscript "c" signifies that this net reabsorption occurs in the collecting ducts (Fig. 8-1). $T^c_{H_2O}$ is equal to $- (C_{H_2O})$.

Summary

Water balance is regulated largely through the intermediation of the antidiuretic hormone (ADH) and the consequent formation of hyperosmotic (concentrated) or hyposmotic (dilute) urine. When a subject is deprived of drinking water, his plasma becomes hyperosmotic. This stimulates the secretion of ADH from the posterior pituitary gland which, by increasing the water permeability of distal tubules and collecting ducts, promotes the reabsorption and hence the conservation of water. Conversely, when a subject imbibes a large amount of water, the consequent dilution of the plasma inhibits the secretion of ADH. This leads to relative water impermeability of the distal tubules and collecting ducts and to the excretion of excess water.

Concentrated urine is formed through passive reabsorption of water by means of the countercurrent mechanism. Countercurrent multiplication of the single effect of reabsorbing Na^+ and Cl^-, virtually without water, from ascending limbs of Henle results in progressive hyperosmolality of the medullary and papillary interstitium. The buildup of this corticopapillary osmotic gradient is aided by the reabsorption of urea from the late portions of the collecting ducts. Dissipation of the gradient by the medullary blood flow is minimized by the countercurrent configuration of the vasa recta, which enables them to function as countercurrent exchangers. In the presence of high concentrations of ADH and resultant high water permeability, water is reabsorbed passively in response to the osmotic gradient between collecting ducts and surrounding interstitium, and hyperosmotic urine is formed.

During formation of dilute urine, the countercurrent mechanism continues to function qualitatively in the same manner. But now, in the absence of ADH, water reabsorption from distal tubules and collecting ducts is minimized despite the existence of osmotic gradients. Consequently, hyposmotic urine is excreted.

The excretion of solute-free water is gauged in relation to the isosmotic plasma that is filtered. When urine is hyposmotic to plasma, relatively more water than solute must have been removed or cleared from the filtered plasma. Hence, under these circumstances the free-water clearance — a misnomer — has a positive sign. When urine is hyperosmotic to plasma, relatively less water than solute must have been removed (or cleared) from the filtered plasma; therefore, under these conditions, C_{H_2O} is negative. Finally, when the urine is isosmotic with plasma, equivalent amounts of solute and water were cleared from the filtered plasma, and C_{H_2O} is zero.

Problem 8-1. Renal handling of salt, water, and urea in varying diuretic states.

The following data were obtained on a healthy medical student, under three conditions: (a) while drinking ad libitum; (b) after 12 hours of thirsting; and (c) within 90 minutes after drinking 1 liter of tap water. Fill in the blanks, and be sure to specify units. Neglect corrections for plasma water and for Donnan distribution.

	$\dot{V}$ (ml/min)	U_{In} (mg/ml)	P_{In} (mg/ml)	GFR	U/P Inulin	Proportion of Filtered Water (i.e., of GFR) Reabsorbed (%)
While drinking ad libitum	1.2	15.8	0.151			
After 12 hours of thirsting	0.75	25.2	0.155			
Within 90 minutes after drinking 1 liter water	15.0	1.23	0.154			

Problem 8-1 continued on pages 142 and 143.

Problem 8-1 *(Cont.)*

	P_{Na} (mEq/L)	Filtered Load of Na	U_{Na} (mEq/L)	Urinary Na Excretion	Proportion of Filtered Na Reabsorbed (%)
While drinking ad libitum	136		128		
After 12 hours of thirsting	144		192		
Within 90 minutes after drinking 1 liter water	134		10.2		

Problem 8-1 *(Cont.)*

	U_{Osm}	P_{Osm}	C_{H_2O}	$T^c_{H_2O}$	$U_{Urea\ N}$[a]	$P_{Urea\ N}$[a]	C_{Urea}	Proportion of Filtered Urea Reabsorbed
	(mOsm/kg)	(mOsm/kg)			(mg/100 ml)			(%)
While drinking ad libitum	663	290			480	12		
After 12 hours of thirsting	1,000	300			720	15		
Within 90 minutes after drinking 1 liter water	100	287			48	10		

[a]Concentrations of urea are usually determined by measuring the amount of nitrogen in urea; hence, the expression *urea nitrogen*. The two nitrogen atoms constitute 28/60 of the urea molecule: $CO(NH_2)_2$. The clearance of urea (C_{Urea}) can be calculated without converting "Urea N" to "Urea," since the conversion factors for $U_{Urea\ N}$ and $P_{Urea\ N}$ cancel out.

Problem 8-2   Normally, in adult man, about 125 ml of plasma H_2O is filtered into Bowman's space each minute. Of this, about 124 ml per minute is reabsorbed. (a) In which nephron segments is the H_2O reabsorbed, and (b) what happens to the H_2O once it has been reabsorbed?

Selected References

General

Adolph, E. F., et al. *Physiology of Man in the Desert.* Interscience, New York, 1947.

Bentley, P. J. *Endocrines and Osmoregulation.* Springer, New York, 1971.

Berliner, R. W., Levinsky, N. G., Davidson, D. G., and Eden, M. Dilution and concentration of the urine and the action of antidiuretic hormone. *Amer. J. Med.* 24:730, 1958.

Dicker, S. E. *Mechanisms of Urine Concentration and Dilution in Mammals.* Williams & Wilkins, Baltimore, 1970.

Gamble, J. L. *Physiological Information Gained from Studies on the Life Raft Ration.* Harvey Lectures, Series XLII, 1946–1947. Science Press, Lancaster, 1947.

Gottschalk, C. W. Micropuncture studies of tubular function in the mammalian kidney. *Physiologist* 4:35, 1961.

Gottschalk, C. W. Osmotic concentration and dilution of the urine. *Amer. J. Med.* 36:670, 1964.

Gottschalk, C. W., and Mylle, M. Micropuncture study of the mammalian urinary concentrating mechanism: Evidence for the countercurrent hypothesis. *Amer. J. Physiol.* 196:927, 1959.

Kuhn, W., and Ryffel, K. Herstellung konzentrierter Lösungen aus verdünnten durch blosse Membranwirkung. Ein Modellversuch zur Funktion der Niere. *Z. Physiol. Chem.* 276:145, 1942.

Marsh, D. J. Osmotic Concentration and Dilution of the Urine. In C. Rouiller and A. F. Muller (Eds.), *The Kidney,* vol. III. Academic, New York, 1971.

This is an excellent general review, which critically discusses unresolved questions about the countercurrent multiplier hypothesis, as well as alternatives to this hypothesis.

Newburgh, J. D. The changes which alter renal osmotic work. *J. Clin. Invest.* 22:439, 1943.

Schmidt-Nielsen, K. *Desert Animals: Physiological Problems of Heat and Water.* Oxford University Press, London, 1964.

Strauss, M. B. *Body Water in Man.* Little, Brown, Boston, 1957.

Ullrich, K. J., Kramer, K., and Boylan, J. W. Present knowledge of the countercurrent system in the mammalian kidney. *Progr. Cardiovasc. Dis.* 3:395, 1961.

Wayner, M. J. (Ed.). *Thirst.* Proceedings of the First International Symposium on Thirst in the Regulation of Body Water. Macmillan, New York, 1964.

Wolf, A. V. *Thirst: Physiology of the Urge To Drink and Problems of Water Lack.* Thomas, Springfield, Ill., 1958.

Part II of this book contains several fascinating accounts of extreme acquisition and deprivation of water.

Countercurrent Multipliers and Exchangers

Black, D. A. K. Renal rete mirabile. *Lancet* 2:1141, 1965.

de Rouffignac, C., and Morel, F. Micropuncture study of water, electrolytes, and urea movements along the loops of Henle in *Psammomys. J. Clin. Invest.* 48:474, 1969.

Jamison, R. L. Micropuncture study of segments of thin loop of Henle in the rat. *Amer. J. Physiol.* 215:236, 1968.

Jamison, R. L. Micropuncture study of superficial and juxtamedullary nephrons in the rat. *Amer. J. Physiol.* 218:46, 1970.

Kokko, J. P. Sodium chloride and water transport in the descending limb of Henle. *J. Clin. Invest.* 49:1838, 1970.

Kuhn, W., Ramel, A., Kuhn, H. J., and Marti, E. The filling mechanism of the swimbladder: Generation of high gas pressures through hairpin countercurrent multiplication. *Experientia* 19:497, 1963.

Marsh, D. J. Solute and water flows in thin limbs of Henle's loop in the hamster kidney. *Amer. J. Physiol.* 218:824, 1970.

Marsh, D. J., and Segel, L. A. Analysis of countercurrent diffusion exchange in blood vessels of the renal medulla. *Amer. J. Physiol.* 221:817, 1971.

Marshall, E. K., Jr. The comparative physiology of the kidney in relation to theories of renal secretion. *Physiol. Rev.* 14:133, 1934.

Peter, K. *Untersuchungen über Bau und Entwickelung der Niere.* Fischer, Jena, 1909.

Scholander, P. F. Secretion of gases against high pressures in the swimbladder of deep sea fishes: II. The rete mirabile. *Biol. Bull.* 107:260, 1954.

Scholander, P. F. The wonderful net. *Sci. Amer.* 196:96, 1957.

Sperber, I. Studies on the mammalian kidney. *Zool. Bid. Uppsala* 22:249, 1944.

Ullrich, K. J. Water Permeability of Different Nephron Segments in the Mammalian Kidney. In K. Thurau and H. Jahrmärker (Eds.), *Renal Transport and Diuretics.* Springer, New York, 1969.

Ullrich, K. J. Permeability Characteristics of the Mammalian Nephron. In J. Orloff and R. W. Berliner (Eds.), *Handbook of Physiology.* Section 8: Renal Physiology. American Physiological Society, Washington, D.C., 1973.

Wirz, H. The location of antidiuretic action in the mammalian kidney. In H. Heller (Ed.), *The Neurohypophysis.* Butterworth, London, 1957.

Wirz, H., Hargitay, B., and Kuhn, W. Lokalisation des Konzentrierungsprozesses in der Niere durch direkte Kryoskopie. *Helv. Physiol. Pharmacol. Acta* 9:196, 1951.

Role of Urea

Bray, G. W., and Preston, A. S. Effect of urea on urine concentration in the rat. *J. Clin. Invest.* 40:1952, 1961.

Gamble, J. L., McKhann, C. F., Butler, A. M., and Tuthill, E. An economy of water in renal function referable to urea. *Amer. J. Physiol.* 109:139, 1934.

Morgan, T., and Berliner, R. W. Permeability of the loop of Henle, vasa recta, and collecting duct to water, urea, and sodium. *Amer. J. Physiol.* 215:108, 1968.

Rabinowitz, L., Thompson, A. B., and Wagman, R. B. Effect of acute urea administration on urinary non-urea solute concentration. *Amer. J. Physiol.* 221:242, 1971.

Schmidt-Nielsen, B. (Ed.). *Urea and the Kidney.* Excerpta Medica Foundation, Amsterdam, 1970.

Schmidt-Nielsen, B., and O'Dell, R. Structure and concentrating mechanism in the mammalian kidney. *Amer. J. Physiol.* 200:1119, 1961.

Truniger, B., and Schmidt-Nielsen, B. Intrarenal distribution of urea and related compounds: Effect of nitrogen intake. *Amer. J. Physiol.* 207:971, 1964.

Ullrich, K. J., Drenckhahn, F. O., and Jarausch, K. H. Untersuchungen zum Problem der Harnkonzentrierung und -verdünnung. *Pflügers Arch. Ges. Physiol.* 261:62, 1955.

Ullrich, K. J., and Jarausch, K. H. Untersuchungen zum Problem der Harnkonzentrierung und -verdünnung. *Pflügers Arch. Ges. Physiol.* 262:537, 1956.

Unresolved Questions

Kokko, J., and Rector, F. C., Jr. Countercurrent multiplication system without active transport in inner medulla. *Kidney Int.* 2:214, 1972.

Kriz, W., and Lever, A. F. Renal countercurrent mechanisms: Structure and function. *Amer. Heart J.* 78:101, 1969.

Marsh, D. J. Osmotic Concentration and Dilution of the Urine. In C. Rouiller and A.F. Muller (Eds.), *The Kidney,* vol. III. Academic, New York, 1971.

This is an excellent general review, which critically discusses unresolved questions about the countercurrent multiplier hypothesis, as well as alternatives to this hypothesis.

Stewart, J., and Valtin, H. Computer simulation of osmotic gradient without active transport in renal inner medulla. *Kidney Int.* 2:264, 1972.

Antidiuretic Hormone (ADH) and Other Hormones

Agus, Z. S., and Goldberg, M. Role of antidiuretic hormone in the abnormal water diuresis of anterior hypopituitarism in man. *J. Clin. Invest.* 50:1478, 1971.

Ahmed, A. B. J., George, B. C., Gonzales-Auvert, C., and Dingman, J. F. Increased plasma arginine vasopressin in clinical adrenocortical insufficiency and its inhibition by glucosteroids. *J. Clin. Invest.* 46:111, 1967.

Berde, B. (Ed.). Neurohypophysial Hormones and Similar Polypeptides. In *Handbook of Experimental Pharmacology,* vol. XXIII. Springer, Berlin, 1968.

A series of authoritative articles, with numerous, useful references. Topics covered include anatomy, chemistry, assays, physiology, pharmacology, and others.

Blaschko, H. K. F., Gregory, R. A., Harris, G. W., and Kenner, G. W. (Organizers). Posterior pituitary hormones and neurophysiology: A discussion on polypeptide hormones. *Proc. Roy. Soc.* Series B. 170:3, 1968.

Gauer, O. H., and Henry, J. P. Circulatory basis of fluid volume control. *Physiol. Rev.* 43:423, 1963.

Gauer, O. H., Henry, J. P., and Behn, C. The regulation of extracellular fluid volume. *Ann. Rev. Physiol.* 32:547, 1970.

Grantham, J. J., and Orloff, J. Effect of prostaglandin E₁ on the permeability response of the isolated collecting tubule to vasopressin, adenosine 3',5'—monophosphate, and theophylline. *J. Clin. Invest.* 47:1154, 1968.

Green, H. H., Harrington, A. R., and Valtin, H. On the role of antidiuretic hormone in the inhibition of acute water diuresis in adrenal insufficiency and the effects of gluco- and mineralocorticoids in reversing the inhibition. *J. Clin. Invest.* 49:1724, 1970.

Handler, J., and Orloff, J. The Mechanism of Action of Antidiuretic Hormone. In J. Orloff and R. W. Berliner

(Eds.), *Handbook of Physiology.* Section 8: Renal Physiology. American Physiological Society, Washington, D.C., 1973.

Jewell, P. A., and Verney, E. B. An experimental attempt to determine the site of neurohypophysial osmoreceptors in the dog. *Phil. Trans. Roy. Soc. London.* Series B. 240:197, 1956–57.

Kleeman, C. R., Czaczkes, J. W., and Cutler, R. Mechanisms of impaired water excretion in adrenal and pituitary insufficiency: IV. Antidiuretic hormone in primary and secondary adrenal insufficiency. *J. Clin. Invest.* 43:1641, 1964.

Knobil, E., and Sawyer, W. H. (Eds.). The Pituitary Gland and Its Neuroendocrine Control, part 1. In *Handbook of Physiology,* vol. 4, sec. 7. American Physiological Society, Washington, D.C., 1974.

Rudinger, J. (Ed.). *Oxytocin, Vasopressin and Their Structural Analogues.* Macmillan, New York, 1964.

Schnermann, J., Valtin, H., Thurau, K., Nagel, W., Horster, M., Fischbach, H., Wahl, M., and Liebau, G. Micropuncture studies on the influence of antidiuretic hormone on tubular fluid reabsorption in rats with hereditary hypothalamic diabetes insipidus. *Pflügers Arch. Ges. Physiol.* 306:103, 1969.

Schwartz, I. L., and Schwartz, W. B. (Eds.). Symposium on antidiuretic hormones. *Amer. J. Med.* 42:651, 1967.

Sieker, H. O., Gauer, O. H., and Henry, J. P. The effect of continuous negative pressure breathing on water and electrolyte excretion by the human kidney. *J. Clin. Invest.* 33:572, 1954.

Starling, E. H., and Verney, E. B. The secretion of urine as studied on the isolated kidney. *Proc. Roy. Soc. London.* Series B. 97:321, 1925.

Ufferman, R. C., and Schrier, R. W. Importance of sodium intake and mineralocorticoid hormone in the impaired water excretion in adrenal insufficiency. *J. Clin. Invest.* 51:1639, 1972.

Valtin, H. Sequestration of urea and nonurea solutes in renal tissues of rats with hereditary hypothalamic diabetes insipidus: Effects of vasopressin and dehydration on the countercurrent mechanism. *J. Clin. Invest.* 45:337, 1966.

Verney, E. B. The antidiuretic hormone and the factors which determine its release. *Proc. Roy. Soc. London.* Series B. 135:25, 1947.

9 : H⁺ Balance

The Problem of Mammalian H⁺ Balance

The pH of the blood of normal man is alkaline, and it is maintained within the small range of about 7.37 to 7.42. A narrow range of pH is essential to normal metabolic function, probably because the activities of protein macromolecules such as enzymes, and elements required for blood clotting and muscle contraction, depend on an optimal pH. The extreme range of plasma pH that is compatible with life is about 7.0 to 7.8.

Despite the essential alkalinity, the mammalian body normally produces large amounts of acid, from two major sources. (1) Some 13,000 to 20,000 mMoles of CO_2 is produced daily as the result of oxidative metabolism; when hydrated, this yields the weak acid, carbonic acid.

$$CO_2 + H_2O \rightleftharpoons H_2CO_3 \rightleftharpoons H^+ + HCO_3^- \qquad (9\text{-}1)$$

Because H_2CO_3 is in equilibrium with a volatile component, CO_2, it is often referred to as a volatile acid. (2) In most western countries, where meat constitutes a large part of the diet, there is also a net daily production of some 40 to 60 mMoles of noncarbonic acids, mainly from protein catabolism. Sulfuric acid is produced through the conversion of sulfur in the amino acid residues, cysteine, cystine, and methionine, as exemplified by the following reaction for methionine:

$$2\,C_5H_{11}NO_2S + 15\,O_2 \rightarrow 4H^+ + 2\,SO_4^= + CO\,(NH_2)_2$$

methionine   urea

$$+ 7\,H_2O + 9\,CO_2 \qquad (9\text{-}2)$$

Formation of phosphoric acid during the catabolism of phospholipids makes a minor contribution to the daily production of noncarbonic acids. Because these acids, unlike H_2CO_3, are not in equilibrium with a volatile component, they are known as nonvolatile, or fixed, acids. (In vegetarians, or in others whose diet consists mainly of vegetables and fruits, the net production of noncarbonic constituents consists of alkalis.)

In certain physiological and pathological states, the production of nonvolatile acids may rise tenfold. Examples include the production of lactic acid during muscular exercise and states of hypoxia, and the production of aceto-acetic acid and β-OH butyric acid during uncontrolled diabetes mellitus.

Thus, the problem of mammalian H^+ balance is the defense of normal alkalinity in the face of a constant onslaught of acid.

In recent years, a number of medical experts have preferred a notation of *hydrogen ion concentration*, $[H^+]$, *rather than pH,* in analyzing acid-base disturbances. Both systems have advantages and disadvantages; one can easily switch from one to the other through the expression

$$pH \simeq - \log [H^+]. \tag{9-3}$$

For the sake of clarity, we shall use only pH in this and the next chapter.

Buffering of Nonvolatile (Fixed) Acids

The very effective defense of alkalinity in a normal dog is illustrated in Figure 9-1. It compares the change in the pH of arterial blood plasma when 156 ml of a 1 N HCl solution was

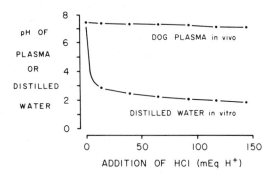

Figure 9-1
An experiment contrasting the effective buffering of HCl in a dog, with the lack of buffering when the same amount of acid is added to distilled water. The pH of the dog's arterial plasma decreased gradually from 7.44 to 7.14; that of unbuffered distilled water dropped precipitously to a level that would be fatal if it occurred in vivo. Redrawn from Pitts, R. F. Harvey Lectures, Series XLVIII, 1952–53. Academic, New York, 1954.

infused intravenously, with the drop in pH when the same amount of acid was gradually added to 11.4 liters of distilled water. This volume of distilled water is about equal to the total body water of the dog. In the dog, the pH dropped from 7.44 to 7.14, a state of severe acidosis but one compatible with survival. In contrast, the addition of just a few milliequivalents of H^+ to unbuffered distilled water lowered the pH to a value that would have been fatal in the animal, and the final level was 1.84. This section deals with the mechanisms that permit such effective buffering in vivo.

First Line of Defense — Fast, Physicochemical Buffering

The following reaction is the prototype for physicochemical buffering:

strong acid + buffer salt ⇌ neutral salt + weak acid   (9-4)

If hydrochloric acid is buffered by the bicarbonate buffer system, the reaction is:

$$H^+ + Cl^- + Na^+ + HCO_3^- \rightleftharpoons Na^+ + Cl^- + H_2CO_3 \qquad (9\text{-}5)$$

Insofar as physicochemical buffering reduces the amount of buffer salt and increases the amount of weak acid, this type of reaction only minimizes, but by no means prevents, a decrease in pH. This point can be illustrated by simple calculations, utilizing the Henderson-Hasselbalch equation as it applies to the bicarbonate system:

$$pH = pK' + \log \frac{[HCO_3^-]}{[H_2CO_3]} \qquad (9\text{-}6)$$

As is shown in Equation 9-1, H_2CO_3 is in equilibrium with dissolved CO_2 in the plasma. In this sense, the dissolved CO_2 is potentially H_2CO_3; the potential supply of H_2CO_3 far exceeds the actual, for at the temperature and ionic concentration of the body fluids, there are about 500 molecules of dissolved CO_2 for every molecule of H_2CO_3. Nevertheless, since H_2CO_3 is in equilibrium with dissolved CO_2, the CO_2 is part of the pool of H_2CO_3 that is available to the organism for buffering. Thus, in a physiological sense, a more meaningful form of the Henderson-Hasselbalch equation is:

$$pH = pK' + \log \frac{[HCO_3^-]}{[\text{dissolved } CO_2 + H_2CO_3]} \qquad (9\text{-}7)$$

The concentration of dissolved CO_2 in plasma is proportional to the partial pressure of CO_2 (P_{CO_2}) in the plasma, which is relatively easy to determine. The proportionality constant for plasma at 38°C, which converts P_{CO_2} in millimeters of mercury (mm Hg) to concentration of dissolved CO_2 expressed as millimoles per liter (mMoles/liter), is 0.03. Thus, ignoring the trace amounts that exist as H_2CO_3, the denominator in Equation 9-7 can be very closely approximated as $P_{CO_2} \cdot 0.03$. For plasma at 38°C, the pK′ (negative logarithm of the apparent dissociation constant) for Equation 9-7 is 6.1. Hence, this equation may be rewritten in a form that is most useful in physiological and clinical practice:

$$pH = 6.1 + \log \frac{[HCO_3^-]}{P_{CO_2} \cdot 0.03} \qquad (9\text{-}8)$$

In this equation, $[HCO_3^-]$ is expressed as mMoles/liter and P_{CO_2} in mm Hg. Substituting values for arterial plasma of man in normal H^+ balance:

$$pH = 6.1 + \log \frac{24 \text{ mMoles/L}}{40 \text{ mm Hg} \cdot 0.03}$$

$$pH = 6.1 + \log \frac{24 \text{ mMoles/L}}{1.2 \text{ mMoles/L}} \qquad (9\text{-}9)$$

$$pH = 6.1 + \log 20$$

$$pH = 7.40$$

If 12 mMoles of HCl were added to each liter of extracellular fluid (which, except for a small Donnan effect, has the same ionic concentrations as plasma), physicochemical buffering would decrease the numerator and increase the denominator by 12 mMoles/liter each, according to the following reaction:

$$12\,H^+ + 12\,Cl^- + 24\,Na^+ + 24\,HCO_3^- \rightleftharpoons 12\,Na^+ + 12\,Cl^-$$

$$+ 12\,H_2CO_3 + 12\,Na^+ + 12\,HCO_3^-$$

$$\Updownarrow \qquad\qquad (9\text{-}10)$$

$$12\,CO_2 + 12\,H_2O$$

If this were to occur in a "closed system" — i.e., without a ventilatory system that can eliminate the newly generated CO_2 — the pH would drop to the fatal level of 6.06.

$$pH = 6.1 + log \frac{12 \text{ mMoles/L}}{1.2 + 12 \text{ mMoles/L}}$$

$$pH = 6.1 + log \frac{12 \text{ mMoles/L}}{13.2 \text{ mMoles/L}}$$

$$pH = 6.06$$

This dire consequence is prevented by the second line of defense, which, like physicochemical buffering, comes into play within seconds or minutes after the administration of HCl.

Second Line of Defense — Fast, Respiratory Component

Actually, virtually all of the H_2CO_3 that was produced through physicochemical buffering is converted to CO_2 and H_2O (Eq. 9-10), and the CO_2 is excreted by the lungs. If all the extra CO_2 were excreted, returning the denominator to 1.2 mMoles/liter, the resulting pH would fall into the range that is compatible with survival.

$$pH = 6.1 + log \frac{12 \text{ mMoles/L}}{1.2 \text{ mMoles/L}}$$

$$pH = 6.1 + log 10$$

$$pH = 7.10$$

Respiratory compensation goes further, however. As a result of the lower pH of the blood, alveolar ventilation is increased, so that alveolar and hence arterial P_{CO_2} are decreased. Consequently the pH is returned toward, but not quite to, the normal value.

$$pH = 6.1 + log \frac{12 \text{ mMoles/L}}{23 \text{ mm Hg} \cdot 0.03}$$

$$pH = 6.1 + log \frac{12 \text{ mMoles/L}}{0.69 \text{ mMoles/L}}$$

$$pH = 7.34$$

Third Line of Defense — Slow, Renal Component

Although respiratory compensation has, within minutes, restored the pH almost to normal, the stores of the main extracellular buffer have been seriously depleted. This fact is reflected in the decrease of the HCO_3^- concentration from 24 to 12 mMoles/liter. Furthermore, some of the added H^+, although admittedly no longer in free solution, still remains within the body as weak acid. Both of these remaining abnormalities are corrected by the kidneys, which excrete H^+ and simultaneously replenish the depleted HCO_3^- stores. This process is a much slower one than the first two lines of defense, requiring hours to days rather than seconds or minutes. How the kidneys accomplish this task is discussed in Chapter 10.

The above is a dramatic example that occurs only under artificial experimental conditions or in disease states. Nevertheless, these are the pathways by which the daily loads of noncarbonic acids are handled. The following quantitative comparison may put the normal, daily challenge from these fixed acids into perspective. An adult person weighing 70 kg has about 14 liters of extracellular fluid (about 20% of body weight; see Fig. 2-1). Hence the addition of 12 mMoles of HCl to each liter of extracellular fluid, as in the example described above, would be a total acid load to an adult human of 168 mMoles (12 mMoles/liter · 14 liters). Not only is the normal daily load of 40 to 60 mMoles of fixed acids merely about one-third of this amount, but also it is released relatively slowly over a 24-hour period, rather than in 1 to 2 hours, as in the above example. If, for the sake of illustration, about one-third of a total load of 48 mMoles were released after each meal, 16 mMoles (48 ÷ 3) would be added to 14 liters of extracellular fluid, i.e., an addition of about 1 mMole per liter of extracellular fluid. Since sulfuric acid is normally the major fixed acid (Eq. 9-2), the quantitative reaction would be as follows:

$$2\,H^+ + SO_4^= + 24\,Na^+ + 24\,HCO_3^- \rightleftharpoons 2\,Na^+ + SO_4^=$$
$$+ 2\,H_2CO_3 + 22\,Na^+ + 22\,HCO_3^-$$
$$\Updownarrow \qquad\qquad\qquad (9\text{-}11)$$
$$2\,CO_2 + 2\,H_2O$$

The resulting pH after physicochemical buffering would be:

$$pH = 6.1 + \log \frac{22 \text{ mMoles/L}}{3.2 \text{ mMoles/L}}$$

$$pH = 6.9$$

After elimination of the extra CO_2 through the lungs, the pH would be:

$$pH = 6.1 + \log \frac{22 \text{ mMoles/L}}{1.2 \text{ mMoles/L}}$$

$$pH = 7.36$$

This might cause only an undetectable increase in alveolar ventilation, thereby restoring the pH to near normal levels. However, what actually happens in a normal individual in the steady state, is that the renal excretion of H^+ and reabsorption of HCO_3^- (Third Line of Defense — see Chap.10), which goes on continually, maintains the arterial plasma concentration of HCO_3^- at about 24 mMoles/liter. Hence, the pH remains normal, as in Equation 9-9.

Buffering of the Volatile Acid, H_2CO_3

At the beginning of this chapter we cited the fact that some 13,000 to 20,000 mMoles of CO_2 is produced daily by an adult person, as the result of metabolic events. This CO_2 is converted by hydration to the weak acid, H_2CO_3 (Eq. 9-1). Normally, elimination of these large amounts of CO_2 by the lungs prevents acidosis (Eq. 9-8). Nevertheless, defense of alkalinity is threatened as the CO_2 is carried in the blood from the cells where it is produced to the lungs where it is excreted. The extremely effective buffering of carbonic acid by the blood is reflected in the fact that the difference in pH between venous blood, which goes to the lungs, and arterial blood, which leaves them, seldom exceeds 0.04 of a pH unit. This section deals with the mechanisms by which carbonic acid is buffered, or in other words, how CO_2 is carried in the blood.

Transport of CO_2 in Blood

The plasma P_{CO_2} at the arterial end of tissue capillaries is about 40 mm Hg. Since the P_{CO_2} is higher in tissue cells that produce CO_2, the gas will diffuse from the tissue cells into the capillary. The chain of events that then occurs is shown in Figure 9-2, and is as follows:

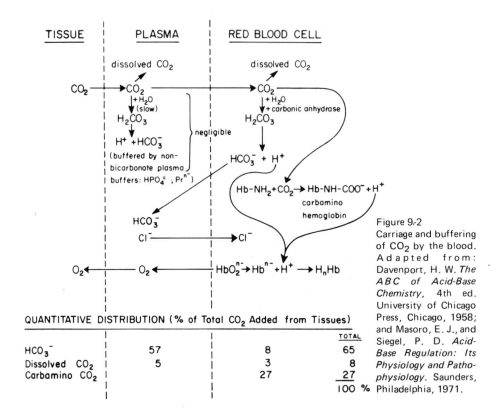

Figure 9-2
Carriage and buffering of CO_2 by the blood. Adapted from: Davenport, H. W. *The ABC of Acid-Base Chemistry*, 4th ed. University of Chicago Press, Chicago, 1958; and Masoro, E. J., and Siegel, P. D. *Acid-Base Regulation: Its Physiology and Pathophysiology.* Saunders, Philadelphia, 1971.

QUANTITATIVE DISTRIBUTION (% of Total CO_2 Added from Tissues)

			TOTAL
HCO_3^-	57	8	65
Dissolved CO_2	5	3	8
Carbamino CO_2		27	27
			100 %

1. Most cell membranes, including those of erythrocytes, are highly permeable to CO_2. Hence CO_2 diffuses not only into the plasma, but also into the erythrocytes. Because there is much carbonic anhydrase in erythrocytes but none in plasma, hydration of CO_2 proceeds much more rapidly within these cells than in the plasma. In fact, the hydration of CO_2 in plasma is negligible; the little bit of H^+ that is formed from this reaction is buffered by the nonbicarbonate buffer anions of plasma, the proteins (Pr^{n-}) and phosphate ($HPO_4^=$).

2. The rapid hydration of CO_2 within the erythrocytes yields HCO_3^-. Most of the newly formed HCO_3^- diffuses into the plasma, and Cl^- shifts into the erythrocytes. In this way, most of the CO_2 that is added to capillary blood is carried to the lungs as HCO_3^- in the plasma. A small portion combines with hemoglobin to form carbamino hemoglobin, and an even smaller amount is carried as dissolved CO_2 within the erythrocytes.

The H⁺ that is formed during the hydration of CO_2 is buffered primarily by hemoglobin. The same is true of the H⁺ that is released during the formation of carbamino hemoglobin.

3. In a normal, resting adult human, every liter of venous blood that goes to the lungs carries about 1.68 mMoles of extra CO_2 for excretion. The quantitative distribution of the various forms in which the added CO_2 is carried is shown at the bottom of Figure 9-2. About 65% of the 1.68 mMoles is carried as HCO_3^-, and the vast majority of this is carried in the plasma, even though virtually all of it was generated within the erythrocytes. The remainder is divided between dissolved CO_2 and carbamino CO_2. Of these, the major portion of dissolved CO_2 is carried in the plasma, whereas practically all the carbamino CO_2 is found in the erythrocytes.

Hemoglobin as a Buffer

Hemoglobin has special attributes as a buffer; these minimize the decrease in pH as CO_2 is added to venous blood. The pH drops from about 7.40 in arterial blood to only about 7.37 in venous blood, rather than to about 7.32, which would be predicted if hemoglobin did not have these special properties. The mechanisms for this effect are shown in Figure 9-3.

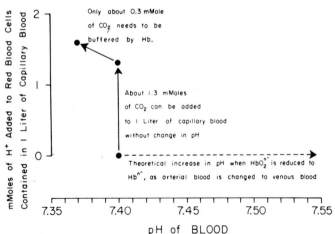

Figure 9-3
The special attributes of hemoglobin as a buffer. The pK' of reduced hemoglobin (Hbⁿ⁻) is higher than that of oxygenated hemoglobin (HbO₂ⁿ⁻). Therefore, hemoglobin becomes a more effective buffer at precisely the moment when CO_2, and hence H⁺, is added from the tissue cells to the blood.

The pK$'$ of oxygenated hemoglobin (HbO_2^{n-}) is lower than the pK$'$ of reduced hemoglobin (Hb^{n-}); i.e., Hb^{n-} is less acidic than HbO_2^{n-}. As blood enters the arteriolar end of tissue capillaries, it gives up O_2 to the cells. The consequent reduction of HbO_2^{n-} to Hb^{n-} *would* cause a tremendous rise in pH were it not for the fact that CO_2, and hence H^+, is simultaneously added to the system. The net result of the change in pK$'$ of hemoglobin is that roughly 1.3 mMoles of CO_2 can be added to each liter of blood as it flows through the tissue capillaries, without changing the pH of that blood. Nearly 95% of the CO_2 that is added to each liter of venous blood, or about 1.6 mMoles of CO_2, is converted to H^+ (Fig. 9-2). Since 1.3 mMoles could be added without a change in pH, only about 0.3 mMole needs to be buffered by Hb^{n-}, and the drop in pH of venous blood is thus minimized.

Concept of Metabolic and Respiratory Disturbances

Primary Disturbances

Inspection of one form of the Henderson-Hasselbalch equation (Eq. 9-8) makes clear that an abnormality of plasma pH can result from a primary deviation of either the $[HCO_3^-]$ or of the P_{CO_2}. Since the concentration of the latter is regulated by the rate of alveolar ventilation, any disturbance in H^+ balance that results from a primary change in P_{CO_2} is called respiratory. Thus, hypoventilation and retention of CO_2 lead to a reduction in pH that is called respiratory acidosis; hyperventilation and a fall in P_{CO_2} lead to a rise in pH that is called respiratory alkalosis. Changes in the concentration of HCO_3^- are brought about most commonly by the net addition or net loss of nonvolatile (fixed) acids or bases, which are derived mainly from metabolic processes. Hence, any abnormality of pH resulting primarily from a change in HCO_3^- is called metabolic. The endogenous production of aceto-acetic acid and β-OH butyric acid in uncontrolled diabetes mellitus leads to metabolic acidosis, while prolonged vomiting with loss of gastric HCl results in metabolic alkalosis.

Thus, there are four primary disturbances of H^+ balance (more often called acid-base balance): (a) respiratory acidosis, (b) respiratory alkalosis, (c) metabolic acidosis, and (d) metabolic alkalosis.

*Mixed
Disturbances*

Sometimes two primary disturbances, usually one respiratory and the other metabolic, occur simultaneously in the same individual. Such patients are said to have "mixed" acid-base disturbances. For example, a patient who manifests alveolar hypoventilation from emphysema may also have an obstructed duodenal ulcer leading to loss of HCl through vomiting. This patient would have a mixed disturbance of respiratory acidosis and metabolic alkalosis. Another patient may have both emphysema with retention of CO_2, and renal failure, which leads to the retention of fixed acids. This patient would have a mixed disturbance of respiratory acidosis and metabolic acidosis.

Since a mixed disturbance usually has a respiratory and a metabolic component, each of which may be acidosis or alkalosis, there are four major mixed disturbances: (a) respiratory acidosis plus metabolic acidosis, (b) respiratory acidosis plus metabolic alkalosis, (c) respiratory alkalosis plus metabolic acidosis, and (d) respiratory alkalosis plus metabolic alkalosis.

*Compensatory
Responses*

Most primary disturbances in H^+ balance tend to elicit a secondary response that partially corrects the pH. In the example cited earlier in this chapter, the addition of HCl led to a decrease in HCO_3^- and hence to metabolic acidosis. This disturbance was largely compensated for by the second line of defense, in which alveolar hyperventilation lowered the P_{CO_2} and thereby adjusted the pH to a near normal value.

This example illustrates two points: (a) that a compensatory response involves the system opposite to the one that caused the primary disturbance (e.g., *metabolic* alkalosis is compensated for by a *respiratory* response, and vice versa) and (b) that compensation shifts the pH *toward* but not to the normal value. Regarding the second point, in the example given earlier in this chapter, respiratory compensation moved the pH to 7.34 but not entirely into the normal range. The reason for this is probably that the compensatory hyperventilation is controlled not only by the pH but also by the P_{CO_2}. The latter declines as alveolar hyperventilation is induced, and the degree of hyperventilation will thus be set at a point where the stimulus to ventilation resulting from the decreased pH will be balanced by the inhibition to respiration resulting from the lowered arterial P_{CO_2}.

Since primary disturbances may be either metabolic or respiratory in origin, and may cause either acidosis or alkalosis, there are four general types of compensatory responses: (1) Metabolic acidosis is compensated for within minutes by alveolar hyperventilation. (2) Metabolic alkalosis may be accompanied by a respiratory compensation that decreases alveolar ventilation, but this response is not invariable. (3) If the primary disturbance is respiratory acidosis, it is usually compensated for by increased renal excretion of H^+ and increased renal reabsorption of HCO_3^-. This response takes days to develop. The mechanisms by which it is accomplished are described in Chapter 10. (4) Finally, respiratory alkalosis is compensated for by a change in the metabolic component of Equation 9-8, namely, by decreased renal excretion of H^+ and decreased renal reabsorption of HCO_3^-.

The Important Buffers of Mammals

Thus far we have spoken almost exclusively about the bicarbonate and the hemoglobin buffer systems. In this section we shall emphasize that the body contains other important buffers, and that all these participate in the regulation of pH.

A buffer is a mixture of either a weak acid and its conjugate base, or of a weak base and its conjugate acid. (Acid is here defined as a H^+ donor and base as a H^+ acceptor.) The buffers of physiological importance in mammals are all of the first type. They have been listed in Figure 9-4. These buffer systems are by no means limited to the plasma. They are found in all phases of the body fluids — plasma, interstitial fluid, intracellular fluid, and bone. The bicarbonate system predominates in plasma and

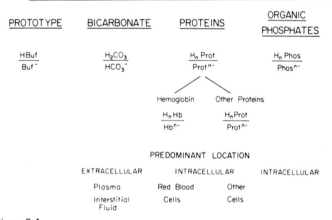

Figure 9-4
The important buffer systems of the mammalian body fluid compartments. The locations refer to quantitative predominance, and are not exclusive except for hemoglobin in erythrocytes. The valence of phosphate is designated as indefinite because it is quantitatively an important chemical buffer mainly within the intracellular fluid, where its valence as organic phosphate is not known.

interstitial fluid, while organic phosphates and proteins (especially hemoglobin) predominate in the intracellular spaces.

The Isohydric Principle

When several buffers exist in a common solution, as in a beaker, all the buffer pairs are in equilibrium with the same concentration of H^+. Expressed in the terminology of the Henderson-Hasselbalch equation, and for plasma — which is a common solution containing the bicarbonate, protein, and phosphate buffer systems — the isohydric principle can be stated as follows:

$$pH = pK_1' + \log \frac{[HCO_3^-]}{[H_2CO_3]} = pK_2' + \log \frac{[HPO_4^=]}{[H_2PO_4^-]} = pK_3' + \log \frac{[Prot^{n-}]}{[H_n Prot]} \qquad (9\text{-}12)$$

This principle has an important application in the analysis of acid-base disturbances, because one can infer the status of most of the body buffer pairs by determining the status of just one of them. In practice, one usually measures two of the three variables of the bicarbonate system, so that the third can easily be calculated (Eq. 9-8). For plasma, which is truly a common solution, knowledge of the bicarbonate system can thus be extended precisely to the phosphate and protein buffer pairs without actually measuring their concentration.

Precise extension to the buffers in the other major fluid compartments is not possible because these compartments are not part of a homogeneous solution in which all the buffers are evenly distributed (Chap. 2). Largely because of the Gibbs-Donnan effect, and partly because of the metabolic production of acids, the pH is considerably lower (perhaps 7.00 or even 6.00) within cells than in the plasma or interstitial fluid. Nevertheless, in many conditions of H^+ imbalance, the isohydric principle can be applied to infer qualitative changes in all or most of the body buffers from knowledge of the bicarbonate system alone. This is permissible because many acid-base disturbances represent relatively chronic situations in which the change in H^+ balance within one fluid compartment has been accompanied by qualitatively similar changes in the other compartments.

Special Attributes of the Bicarbonate System

We have already reviewed the special properties of hemoglobin that render it extraordinarily suitable for buffering the H^+ that is formed when CO_2 is added to venous blood. In turn, the bicarbonate system has special attributes for buffering noncarbonic acids. Titration curves for the bicarbonate and inorganic phosphate buffers, which are found in plasma and interstitial fluid, are shown in Figure 9-5. Several points should be noted: (a) the pK' is numerically equal to the pH existing when the weak acid and its conjugate base each comprise 50% of the total concentration of that particular buffer; (b) the change in pH per quantum of H^+ or OH^- added is least in the linear portion of each titration curve; and (c) this linear portion of most effective chemical buffering extends roughly 1.0 pH unit to either side of the pK' — from pH of about 5.1 to 7.1 for the bicarbonate system, and from about 5.8 to 7.8 for phosphate. In other words, in the range of plasma pH that is compatible with survival (about 7.00 to 7.80), phosphate is a far more effective chemical buffer than is the bicarbonate system. Nevertheless, bicarbonate plays a much more important physiological role as an extracellular buffer than does phosphate.

The reason for the seeming paradox is not only that the extracellular concentration of bicarbonate (about 24 mMoles/liter) is so much higher than that of phosphate (1 to 2 mMoles/liter; Fig. 2-2), but also, and more importantly, that bicarbonate has certain physiological properties that make it a uniquely effective buffer. The central property is that carbonic acid is in equilibrium with volatile CO_2, which can be rapidly

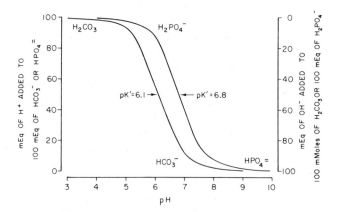

Figure 9-5
Titration curves for the bicarbonate and inorganic phosphate buffers in a closed system. Under these conditions, when the concentration of H_2CO_3 cannot be kept low through elimination of CO_2, the bicarbonate system is a less effective buffer than phosphate. It is mainly because CO_2 can normally be eliminated by the lungs that the bicarbonate system is such an efficient physiological buffer. Modified from Pitts, R. F. *Physiology of the Kidney and Body Fluids*, 2d ed. Year Book, Chicago, 1968.

excreted or retained by the lungs (see the Second Line of Defense earlier in this chapter). Furthermore, both the weak acid and the conjugate base of the bicarbonate buffer system are more abundantly available from daily metabolic processes than are those of any other buffer system.

Utilization of the Various Buffers

Addition of Strong Acid. Earlier in this chapter when we described the buffering of nonvolatile (fixed) acids (i.e., acids other than carbonic acid), we limited the analysis to the bicarbonate buffer system in plasma. This simplification was not inaccurate, since an acid that is infused intravenously will initially have its impact on the plasma. The simplification, however, presented an incomplete picture in that it did not include the participation of the other buffer systems of the body. The total picture is presented in Figure 9-6, which indicates not only the time course for distribution of a fixed acid throughout the body fluid compartments, but also the quantitative contribution of the major buffers.

Figure 9-6 is based on experimental work in dogs that were given intravenous infusions of hydrochloric acid over periods of 1.5 to 3 hours. Within seconds to minutes, the acid is being handled by the various buffers of the blood. In the plasma, this process involves mainly the bicarbonate system, because its ionic concentration in plasma is so much greater than that of the proteins and inorganic phosphate (Fig. 2-2), and because CO_2, which is formed in the buffering reaction, is quickly excreted via the lungs. The acid also quickly enters the erythrocytes, where it is buffered primarily by hemoglobin; bicarbonate, and to an even lesser extent organic phosphates, within erythrocytes contribute a little bit to the buffering. A small amount of the acid is buffered in the plasma, by bicarbonate that was derived from the erythrocytes through an exchange of Cl^- for HCO_3^-.

As soon as the HCl is infused into the plasma, it begins to enter the interstitial compartment. Although it takes about one-half hour for the acid to be evenly distributed between the plasma and interstitial fluid, the latter actually contributes more to the total buffering because its volume is about 4 times greater than that of plasma (see Fig. 2-1). Again, inorganic phosphate in the interstitium also participates, but to a negligible extent because its concentration in interstitial fluid is so low.

Several hours elapse before the acid is evenly distributed throughout the intracellular compartment. Nevertheless, the contribution of the intracellular buffers is great. Utilization of

ON DAY OF ACID INFUSION

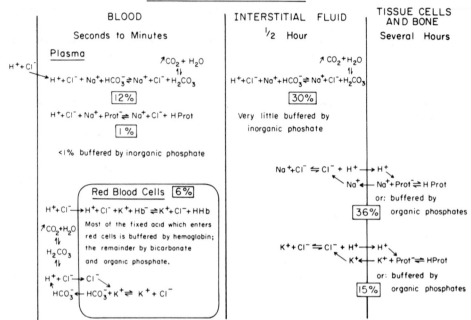

24 HOURS AFTER INFUSING ACID

About 25% of acid load has been excreted in the urine as titratable acid and NH_4^+ (see Chapter 10). Extracellular pH and ionic composition are nearly normal; therefore, 75% of the administered acid must be sequestered and buffered in tissue cells and bone.

SECOND TO SIXTH DAYS AFTER INFUSING ACID

The remaining 75% of the administered acid is slowly released from tissue cells and bone, and excreted in the urine.

Figure 9-6
Handling of the fixed acid, HCl, by intact dogs. For the sake of clarity, polyvalent anions such as proteins and hemoglobin, have been drawn with a single negative sign. A slanted arrow next to CO_2 indicates that the CO_2 is quickly excreted through the lungs. The percentages enclosed in rectangles indicate the approximate proportion of the total acid load that is buffered by each mechanism. Data from: Swan, R. C., and Pitts, R. F. *J. Clin. Invest.* 34:205, 1955; Yoshimura, H., et al. *Jap. J. Physiol.* 11:109, 1961; Pitts, R. F. *Physiology of the Kidney and Body Fluids,* 2d ed. Year Book, Chicago, 1968; and Masoro, E. J., and Siegel, P. D. *Acid-Base Regulation: Its Physiology and Pathophysiology.* Saunders, Philadelphia, 1971.

these buffers — mainly proteins and organic phosphates — is accomplished by exchange of extracellular H^+ for either intra-cellular Na^+ or intracellular K^+. Some of the Na^+ probably comes from the apatite of bone, and the H^+ that is exchanged for this Na^+ enters into a chemical reaction with the apatite, finally being incorporated into HCO_3^-. The involvement of bone in buffering is probably much more important during chronic disturbances of acid-base balance than during the relatively acute disturbance illustrated in Figure 9-6.

The relative quantitative contributions of the various buffers is indicated by the boxes in Figure 9-6, which give the percentage of the total acid load that is handled by each mechanism. It is clear that less than 15% is buffered in the plasma, and less than 20% by whole blood. In fact, the largest proportion, or about one-half of the administered acid, is buffered in the intracellular compart-ment.

Although buffering of the acid has minimized changes in pH, full restoration to the normal state must await excretion of the acid load in the urine. This occurs during the ensuing six days. By the second day after the infusion, about 25% of the acid has been excreted, and both the pH and ionic composition of the extracellular fluids have returned to near normal values. It follows that 75% of the acid load must now reside within the cells and bone, where it is buffered. This remaining acid is slowly released into the extracellular fluids and excreted by the kidneys during the second to sixth days after the acid was given.

Addition of Strong Alkali. When strong base such as sodium bicarbonate is infused intravenously, or HCl is eliminated as by vomiting, the chain of events is similar to that discussed above, except that the reactions go in the opposite direction. There is a very significant participation by the intracellular buffers, and the time course for the utilization of the various buffers is similar to that shown in Figure 9-6. Three differences should be noted, however: (a) respiratory compensation — i.e., alveolar hypo-ventilation due to an increase in pH — does not invariably occur and is frequently not as effective in metabolic alkalosis as in metabolic acidosis; (b) lactic acid moves out of skeletal muscle cells, to buffer the base in the extracellular fluid; and (c) the renal excretion of sodium bicarbonate occurs more rapidly than does the renal excretion of H^+.

Addition of Carbonic Acid. Carbonic acid is produced through the hydration of CO_2 (Eq. 9-1). If excess CO_2 is produced endogenously and there is no disorder of respiration, the excess CO_2 is quickly excreted through the lungs by the mechanisms outlined earlier in this chapter and shown in Figure 9-2. If, however, CO_2 is either added from an external source as by breathing a gas mixture containing 5% CO_2, or CO_2 accumulates because of some disorder of respiration, there is a net addition of carbonic acid to the body. The chain of events that is set into motion under these circumstances is shown in Figure 9-7.

The first important point to recognize is that carbonic acid cannot be buffered by the bicarbonate buffer system. The reason for this is evident from the following reaction:

$$\uparrow CO_2 + H_2O \rightleftharpoons H_2CO_3 \rightleftharpoons H^+ + HCO_3^- \qquad (9\text{-}13)$$

$$\Updownarrow + Na^+ + Buf^-$$

$$H\,Buf + Na^+ + HCO_3^-$$

The arrow in front of the CO_2 indicates that the initial event is the addition of CO_2; hence the reaction is being driven to the right and it cannot proceed to the left as it would have to if the H^+ were to be buffered by HCO_3^-. Instead, the H^+ must be buffered by the nonbicarbonate buffers (proteins and phosphates), here termed Buf^-. As is shown in Figure 9-4, the only buffer of quantitative importance in the extracellular fluid is the bicarbonate system. It follows, then, that very little of the added carbonic acid — in fact less than 5% (Fig. 9-7) — can be buffered in the extracellular compartment, i.e., in the plasma and interstitial fluid.

A second important distinction between the addition of a strong acid and the addition of carbonic acid lies in the time required for the acid load to be distributed throughout the major fluid compartments. This process takes hours for a strong acid (Fig. 9-6), whereas it occurs within minutes for H_2CO_3 (Fig. 9-7), because CO_2 diffuses so readily across both the vascular endothelium and the cell membrane.

Hemoglobin, of course, is the most abundant nonbicarbonate buffer in blood (Fig. 9-4). Consequently, a large proportion of the added H_2CO_3 is buffered by the various mechanisms outlined in Figure 9-2. Since CO_2 diffuses so easily across cell membranes, the reactions in erythrocytes occur within seconds to minutes after the onset of the disturbance. During this time, a relatively normal plasma pH will be preserved. However, since H_2CO_3 is simultaneously being formed in the interstitial compartment, where it initially cannot be buffered, there will then ensue a

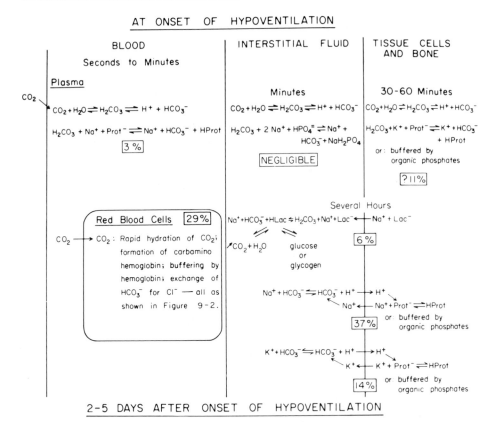

AT ONSET OF HYPOVENTILATION

BLOOD | **INTERSTITIAL FLUID** | **TISSUE CELLS AND BONE**

Figure 9-7

Events that follow the retention of CO_2 (and hence the addition of H_2CO_3) due to prolonged alveolar hypoventilation. For the sake of clarity, polyvalent protein anions have been written with a single negative sign. The approximate proportion of the total acid load that is buffered by each mechanism is indicated by the percentages in the rectangles; the figure of 11% is uncertain. Data adapted from: Giebisch, G., et al. *J. Clin. Invest.* 34:231, 1955; Pitts, R. F. *Physiology of the Kidney and Body Fluids,* 2d ed. Year Book, Chicago, 1968; and Masoro, E. J., and Siegel, P. D. *Acid-Base Regulation: Its Physiology and Pathophysiology.* Saunders, Philadelphia, 1971.

dramatic drop in plasma pH as the H^+ is distributed evenly throughout the plasma and interstitial fluid. It takes several hours before the intracellular nonhemoglobin buffers make a quantitatively significant contribution to handling the H_2CO_3 that was formed in the extracellular space. This is accomplished mainly by exchange of H^+ for Na^+ and H^+ for K^+ across cell membranes, and to a lesser extent by lactate moving out of cells. The H_2CO_3 that is formed within cells is buffered by the nonbicarbonate buffers in these cells.

Thus, since H_2CO_3 cannot be buffered by the bicarbonate system, all but 3% of the added acid load is buffered either within cells (erythrocytes, tissue cells, and bone) or through buffers (lactate) derived from cells.

As was the case after the addition of strong acid, so here too the renal response is a relatively slow one requiring days before a new equilibrium state is reached. In this connection, a third difference between the addition of a strong acid and the addition of H_2CO_3 should be noted. The events occurring on the day of adding strong acid (Fig. 9-6) include the rapid second line of defense (see earlier in this chapter), in which the excretion of CO_2 "adjusts" the denominator of the Henderson—Hasselbalch equation. Consequently, a near normal plasma pH is attained quickly. However, when the primary acid-base disturbance is respiratory (i.e., when the initial change is in the denominator of the Henderson-Hasselbalch equation), the events occurring at the onset are limited to chemical buffering (Fig. 9-7), and compensatory "adjustment" of the numerator must await the much slower renal process. Hence, primary respiratory disturbances are accompanied by relatively marked deviations of pH during the first few days, and a near normal pH is attained only after a number of days.

Deficit of Carbonic Acid. The responses that set in when alveolar hyperventilation reduces the CO_2, and hence H_2CO_3, are analogous to those depicted in Figure 9-7, except that the reactions proceed in the opposite direction.

Summary

Every day, normal man produces large quantities of acid. In an adult, this amounts to at least 13,000 mMoles of H_2CO_3 derived from oxidative metabolism, and a net production of about 50 mMoles of noncarbonic acids if he is eating meat. Despite these large loads of acid, man maintains an alkaline plasma pH, which is crucial to his survival.

H_2CO_3, which is normally derived through the hydration of metabolically generated CO_2, is quickly excreted through the lungs as CO_2; it is therefore called a volatile acid. H_2CO_3 can be transported from the cells to the lungs, with minimal reduction in the pH of blood, because of the special property of hemoglobin as a buffer. This property derives from the fact that reduced hemoglobin is a weaker acid than oxygenated hemoglobin. Hence, as capillary blood releases O_2, it can take up a great deal of CO_2 without any change in pH.

Acids other than H_2CO_3 do not have a volatile component; they are therefore known as nonvolatile, or "fixed," acids.

Normally, such acids are derived from the catabolism primarily of proteins, and to a lesser extent of phospholipids. Acid-base balance in the face of these acids is preserved by three lines of defense: (a) physicochemical buffering, which begins within seconds after introducing the acid; (b) adjustments in alveolar ventilation, which occur within seconds or minutes; and (c) renal excretion of H^+ and renal reabsorption of HCO_3^-, which may take days to come to completion. The bicarbonate buffer system is especially effective in handling excesses or deficits of fixed acids because: (a) it has a volatile component, CO_2, which can be regulated by changes in alveolar ventilation and (b) the substrates of this buffer system are readily available from metabolic processes.

Disturbances of H^+ balance may be either metabolic or respiratory in origin. The first will cause a deviation in the numerator of the Henderson-Hasselbalch equation (Eq. 9-8), which will tend to shift the pH in either an acid or an alkaline direction; the second will lead to a deviation in the denominator, which likewise may shift the pH in either direction. In most instances, a primary disturbance of one origin (i.e., metabolic or respiratory) is accompanied by a second response of opposite origin (i.e., respiratory or metabolic, respectively), which restores the plasma pH toward normal. When primary disturbances of metabolic and respiratory origin occur simultaneously in the same individual, then the resulting state is known as a mixed disturbance.

A load of acid or of alkali calls into play not only the buffers of the plasma, but also those of interstitial fluid, cells, and bone. Roughly 50% of fixed acid is buffered within cells. In contrast, more than 95% of an excess or deficit of carbonic acid is buffered intracellularly; this is so because H_2CO_3 cannot be buffered by the bicarbonate system, which is overwhelmingly the predominant buffer of extracellular fluid, i.e., the plasma and interstitium.

The isohydric principle states that all buffer pairs in a common solution are in equilibrium with the same H^+ concentration. The various body fluid compartments do not represent a common solution. Nevertheless, the principle can be applied in most equilibrium states, to assess the approximate status of all buffers in the body. Most disturbances of H^+ balance result in a new equilibrium state (steady state), in which the changes in all body buffers are qualitatively similar. Hence, in relatively chronic acid-base disturbances, analysis of the bicarbonate buffer system in plasma may be extended to gain some knowledge about the other buffers.

Problem 9-1. The data below were obtained on each of four patients. Complete the analysis of the acid-base status of each patient by filling in the blank spaces.

Normal arterial values: pH = 7.37 to 7.42; $[HCO_3^-]$ = 23 to 25 mMoles/L; P_{CO_2} = 38 to 42 mm Hg.

Cause of the Disturbance	Arterial Plasma			Type of Disturbance
	pH	P_{CO_2} (mm Hg)	$[HCO_3^-]$ (mM/L)	
Prolonged vomiting	7.55	44		
Ingestion of $NH_4 Cl^a$		28	10	
Hysterical hyperventilation	7.57		21	
Heroin poisoning	7.07	99		

[a]The net effect of ingesting NH_4Cl is the addition of hydrochloric acid.

$$2NH_4Cl + CO_2 \rightarrow 2H^+ + 2Cl^- + H_2O + \underset{\text{urea}}{CO(NH_2)_2}$$

Appendix *The pH-HCO₃⁻ Diagram*

There are many graphical depictions of the Henderson-Hasselbalch equation. For several reasons, I have avoided the use of such diagrams: they add no new concepts; they tend to promote an "automatic" usage without a full understanding of the dynamics of acid-base balance; and, in clinical situations, such automatic usage can lead to errors in therapy. Nevertheless, beginning students have found that at least one type of graph, the pH-HCO₃⁻ diagram, has helped them to clarify a number of basic concepts in acid-base balance, particularly at a qualitative level. The diagram is therefore presented here — with the admonition, however, that it does not always portray an accurate *quantitative* assessment for all body buffers, especially in chronic respiratory disturbances.

Construction of the Diagram. pH is plotted on the abscissa, against the plasma HCO₃⁻ concentration on the ordinate, as in Figure 9-8. The basis for the diagram is the Henderson-Hasselbalch equation, and the form used is the one given in the text as Equation 9-8:

$$pH = 6.1 + \log \frac{[HCO_3{}^-]}{P_{CO_2} \cdot 0.03} \tag{9-8}$$

If the normal values for arterial plasma given in Problem 9-1 are used, the solid dot in Figure 9-8a denotes the normal state of H⁺ balance. The P_{CO_2} at this point will be 40 mm Hg. If this value is held constant while the plasma HCO₃⁻ concentration is varied, the above equation yields certain values for pH. For example, if the HCO₃⁻ concentration is 12 mMoles/liter, then

$$pH = 6.1 + \log \frac{12 \text{ mMoles/L}}{40 \text{ mm Hg} \cdot 0.03}$$

$$pH = 6.1 + \log \frac{12}{1.2}$$

$$pH = 6.1 + \log 10$$

$$pH = 7.1$$

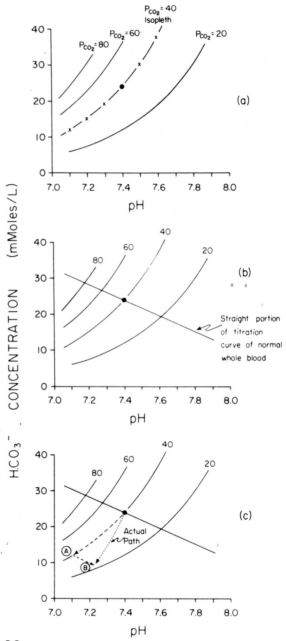

Figure 9-8
Graphical depiction of the Henderson-Hasselbalch equation as the
pH-HCO$_3^-$ diagram. In (a), P$_{CO2}$ isopleths were obtained by substituting
various values for plasma HCO$_3^-$ concentration at constant P$_{CO2}$. The
straight line in (b) represents the CO$_2$ titration curve for normal whole
blood; the slope of this line therefore determines the changes in pH and in
plasma HCO$_3^-$ concentration that take place as CO$_2$ is added to or
subtracted from normal blood. The dynamics involved in the development
of primary metabolic acidosis are portrayed in (c). Slightly modified from
Davenport, H. W. *The ABC of Acid-Base Chemistry,* 4th ed. University of
Chicago Press, Chicago, 1958.

Different values for HCO_3^- concentration when the P_{CO_2} is 40 mm Hg, will yield the pH values set forth below.

P_{CO_2} (mm Hg)	$[HCO_3^-]$ (mM/L)	pH
40	37.9	7.60
40	30.1	7.50
40	24.0	7.40
40	19.1	7.30
40	15.1	7.20
40	12.0	7.10

These points are plotted as "X" in Figure 9-8a. Since all the points that fall on the resulting curve correspond to a P_{CO_2} of 40 mm Hg, the curve is called an isopleth. Isopleths for P_{CO_2} values of 80, 60, and 20 mm Hg have been constructed in a similar manner.

If CO_2 is added to normal blood, the concentrations of H^+ and of HCO_3^- increase (Eq. 9-13). The extent to which they increase — or, phrased differently, the extent to which the pH falls and the plasma HCO_3^- concentration increases — will depend on the nonbicarbonate buffers in blood, i.e., mainly on the concentration of hemoglobin (Fig. 9-2). For example, if the P_{CO_2} of normal blood is raised from 40 to 60 mm Hg, the resulting combination of pH and HCO_3^- concentration must be such that it satisfies the Henderson-Hasselbalch equation, and the new point obviously must fall on the $P_{CO_2} = 60$ mm Hg isopleth. Just where on this curve it falls is determined mainly by the hemoglobin concentration. The same arguments apply to locating the new points when the P_{CO_2} is raised to 80 mm Hg or lowered to 20 mm Hg, or in fact to any new P_{CO_2}. The straight line in Figure 9-8b connects all such points when the P_{CO_2} of normal blood is varied. The slope of the line thus reflects the buffer value of whole blood; it may be drawn here as a straight line because in this range of pH, the titration curve of hemoglobin approximates a straight line (Fig. 9-5).

Thus, the diagram in Figure 9-8b is an accurate portrayal of the Henderson-Hasselbalch equation as it pertains to *normal whole blood*. The diagram can therefore be used to show the changes that occur during primary acid-base disturbances in normal individuals. To illustrate this usage, let us reconsider the example cited earlier in this chapter, where 12 mMoles of HCl were added to each liter of extracellular fluid — i.e., an example of primary metabolic acidosis.

As was shown in Equation 9-10, the added HCl is buffered mainly by $NaHCO_3$. The extra CO_2 that is thereby generated is immediately eliminated through the lungs. If this were all there is to the second line of defense, the P_{CO_2} would remain at 40 mm Hg, and the resulting pH of 7.10 would be reached along the P_{CO_2} = 40 mm Hg isopleth; this is shown by the arrow with the dashed line going to point A in Figure 9-8c. Respiratory compensation, however, lowers the P_{CO_2} — in the example given earlier — to 23 mm Hg (see p. 153). As CO_2 is added to or subtracted from blood, it is buffered by the nonbicarbonate buffers. Hence, the arrow with the dashed line going from point A to point B runs parallel to the titration curve for whole blood. Equation 9-13 shows that as CO_2 is removed from the body, H^+ is liberated from the nonbicarbonate buffers, and in the process, the concentration of HCO_3^- is decreased:

$$\downarrow CO_2 + H_2O \rightleftharpoons H_2CO_3 \rightleftharpoons H^+ + HCO_3^- \qquad (9\text{-}13)$$

$$\Updownarrow + Na^+ + Buf^-$$

$$H\,Buf + Na^+ + HCO_3^-$$

(The downward arrow in front of CO_2 indicates that CO_2 is decreased, so that the reaction is driven to the left.) For the sake of clarity, this effect of titration of nonbicarbonate buffers on the concentration of HCO_3^- was omitted in the earlier discussion (see p. 153); the pH of 7.23 at point B is therefore lower than the previously calculated value of 7.34, when the HCO_3^- concentration was assumed to remain stable as P_{CO_2} was lowered.

Of course, metabolic acidosis does not develop in gross, sequential steps, as to point A and then to point B; rather, the actual path is a composite of small changes that occur simultaneously, shown in Figure 9-8c by the arrow with the dotted line. Restoration to the normal state involves the renal excretion of H^+ and the renal replenishment of HCO_3^-, which returns the HCO_3^- concentration to 24 mMoles/liter and the pH to 7.40. This process, the third line of defense (see p. 154), is described in Chapter 10; in Figure 9-8c, it would follow the actual path from point B to the black dot.

Problem 9-2 By means of a similar analysis as that just outlined for metabolic acidosis, trace on a pH-HCO$_3$⁻ diagram the steps involved in the development of: respiratory acidosis; metabolic alkalosis; and respiratory alkalosis. Locate on a pH-HCO$_3$⁻ diagram, the approximate position of points that would represent the following mixed disturbances of H⁺ balance: respiratory acidosis plus metabolic acidosis; respiratory acidosis plus metabolic alkalosis; respiratory alkalosis plus metabolic acidosis; and respiratory alkalosis plus metabolic alkalosis.

Selected References

General

Bittar, E. E. *Cell pH.* Butterworth, Washington, D.C., 1964.

Christensen, H. N. *Body Fluids and the Acid-Base Balance.* Saunders, Philadelphia, 1964.

Davenport, H. W. *The ABC of Acid-Base Chemistry,* 4th ed. University of Chicago Press, Chicago, 1958.

Henderson, L. J. *Blood: A Study in General Physiology.* Yale University Press, New Haven, 1928.

Masoro, E. J., and Siegel, P. D. *Acid-Base Regulation: Its Physiology and Pathophysiology.* Saunders, Philadelphia, 1971.

Nahas, G. G. (Ed.). Current concepts of acid-base measurement. *Ann. N.Y. Acad. Sci.* 133:1, 1966.

Pitts, R. F. *Physiology of the Kidney and Body Fluids,* 2d ed. Year Book, Chicago, 1968.

Rector, F. C., Jr. (Ed.). Symposium on acid-base homeostasis. *Kidney Int.* 1:273, 1972.

    This recent review is up to date and includes authoritative articles on the following: buffering mechanisms; metabolic alkalosis; renal acidosis; metabolic consequences of acid-base disturbances; pH of the cerebrospinal fluid; and other topics.

Robin, E. D., Bromberg, P. A., and Cross, C. E. Some aspects of the evolution of vertebrate acid-base regulation. *Yale J. Biol. Med.* 41:448, 1969.

Waddell, W. J., and Bates, R. B. Intracellular pH. *Physiol. Rev.* 49:285, 1969.

Winters, R. W., and Dell, R. B. Regulation of Acid-Base Equilibrium. In W. S. Yamamoto and J. R. Brobeck (Eds.), *Physiological Controls and Regulations.* Saunders, Philadelphia, 1965.

Winters, R. W., Engel, K., and Dell, R. B. *Acid-Base Physiology in Medicine: A Self-Instruction Program.* London, Cleveland. 1967.

Buffering

Bergstrom, W. H., and Wallace, W. M. Bone as a sodium and potassium reservoir. *J. Clin. Invest.* 33:867, 1954.

German, B., and Wyman, J., Jr. The titration curves of oxygenated and reduced hemoglobin. *J. Biol. Chem.* 117:533, 1937.

Giebisch, G., Berger, L., and Pitts, R. F. The extrarenal response to acute acid-base disturbances of respiratory origin. *J. Clin. Invest.* 34:231, 1955.

Lennon, E. J., and Lemann, J. Defense of hydrogen ion concentration in chronic metabolic acidosis. *Ann. Intern. Med.* 65:265, 1966.

Pitts, R. F. *Mechanisms for Stabilizing the Alkaline Reserves of the Body.* The Harvey Lectures, Series XLVIII. Academic, New York, 1954.

Swan, R. C., Axelrod, D. R., Seip, M., and Pitts, R. F. Distribution of sodium bicarbonate infused into nephrectomized dogs. *J. Clin. Invest.* 34:1795, 1955.

Swan, R. C., and Pitts, R. F. Neutralization of infused acid by nephrectomized dogs. *J. Clin. Invest.* 34:205, 1955.

Tobin, R. B. Plasma, extracellular and muscle electrolyte responses to acute metabolic acidosis. *Amer. J. Physiol.* 186:131, 1956.

Yoshimura, H., Fujimoto, M., Okumura, O., Sugimoto, J., and Kuwada, T. Three-step-regulation of acid-base balance in body fluid after acid load. *Jap. J. Physiol.* 11:109, 1961.

Primary Disturbances

Goodman, A. D., Lemann, J., Jr., Lennon, E. J., and Relman, A. S. Production, excretion, and net balance of fixed acid in patients with renal acidosis. *J. Clin. Invest.* 44:495, 1965.

Lemann, J., Jr., Lennon, E. J., Goodman, A. D., Litzow, J. R., and Relman, A. S. The net balance of acid in subjects given large loads of acid or alkali. *J. Clin. Invest.* 44:507, 1965.

Polak, A., Haynie, G. D., Hays, R. M., and Schwartz, W. B. Effects of chronic hypercapnia on electrolyte and acid-base equilibrium: I. Adaptation. *J. Clin. Invest.* 40:1223, 1961.

Schwartz, W. B., Hays, R. M., Polak, A., and Haynie, G. D. Effects of chronic hypercapnia on electrolyte and acid-base equilibrium: II. Recovery, with special reference to the influence of chloride intake. *J. Clin. Invest.* 40:1238, 1961.

10 : Renal Excretion of H^+ and Conservation of HCO_3^-

Role of Kidneys in H^+ Balance

It is clear from Chapter 9 that the maintenance of a normal plasma pH depends on the preservation of a normal *ratio* between the weak acid and conjugate base components of each of the body buffers. By the isohydric principle (Eq. 9-12), these ratios can be determined precisely for all plasma buffers, from knowledge of the bicarbonate buffer system in plasma. Except for the slight correction necessitated by the Gibbs-Donnan effect, the plasma bicarbonate system will also reflect the ratio of all interstitial buffers; and as stated previously, in the steady state of most acid-base disturbances, any change in the plasma bicarbonate system will be accompanied by qualitatively similar changes of the intracellular buffers. It thus follows that regulating the ratio of the concentration of HCO_3^- to that of H_2CO_3 (or more precisely, of P_{CO_2}) in plasma, will tend to regulate the ratio of all other buffer pairs.

The weak acid component of the plasma bicarbonate buffer system is regulated as P_{CO_2} through alveolar ventilation (Eq. 9-8). Preservation of the conjugate base, HCO_3^-, is accomplished through the kidneys. This task involves two processes: (a) the reabsorption of virtually all the HCO_3^- that is filtered and (b) the reclamation of the HCO_3^- that was consumed in buffering fixed acids (Eq. 9-11). In the latter process, the H^+ ions of fixed acids that were incorporated into weak buffer acids are excreted by the kidneys. The combination of renal replenishment of HCO_3^- stores and renal excretion of the H^+ of fixed acids was described in Chapter 9 as the Third Line of Defense.

Reabsorption of Filtered HCO_3^-

Like Na^+ and other small solutes, so HCO_3^- is freely filtered by the glomeruli. As is shown in Table 1-1, the daily filtered load of HCO_3^- in an adult human amounts to about 4,500 mEq. If even a very small portion of this were excreted in the urine, the normal stores of this important buffer base would be quickly exhausted. This eventuality is prevented by avid tubular reabsorption of

HCO_3^-, which normally amounts to more than 99.9% of the filtered load (Table 1-1).

Mechanism for Reabsorption of Filtered HCO_3^-

The classic studies of R. F. Pitts and his colleagues showed conclusively that acid can be secreted by the renal tubules. They reasoned that the source of this acid must be largely or exclusively carbonic acid, and they strengthened this thesis by demonstrating that inhibition of the enzyme, carbonic anhydrase (as by administering the compound, acetazolamide), greatly reduced or abolished the amount of acid that could be secreted. They suggested, furthermore, that acid was secreted in the form of H^+ ion in exchange for Na^+, rather than as molecular acid or through some other means. Evidence that the bulk of HCO_3^- reabsorption occurs by a mechanism of H^+ secretion came 20 years later, following a suggestion by M. Walser and G. H. Mudge, and the micropuncture experiments of F. C. Rector, Jr., N. W. Carter, and D. W. Seldin. Figure 10-1 thus rests on experimental observations; nevertheless, it must be cautioned that some parts of the outline have not been fully proved (e.g., Na^+-H^+ exchange).

Within the tubular cell, the hydration of CO_2 is catalyzed by carbonic anhydrase (C.A.). The source of the CO_2 is threefold: (a) oxidative metabolism of the renal cell, (b) peritubular blood, and (c) CO_2 generated within the tubular lumen. The H^+ that is produced in the hydration reaction is secreted into the tubular

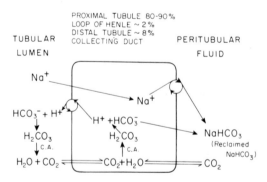

Figure 10-1
Mechanism for the reabsorption of filtered HCO_3^-. C.A. stands for carbonic anhydrase; in the proximal tubule, but not in the distal, tubular fluid is exposed to this enzyme. The percentages indicate the proportion of the filtered HCO_3^- that is reabsorbed in each of the nephron segments. In normal man producing a net amount of fixed acid, virtually all the filtered HCO_3^- is conserved through reabsorption.

lumen; consideration of the transepithelial electrochemical potential difference makes clear that this must be at least in part an active transport process in the proximal tubule, although the mode of transport in more distal nephron segments has not been defined. In the tubular lumen, the secreted H^+ combines with filtered HCO_3^- to form H_2O and CO_2. Because proximal tubular fluid is exposed to carbonic anhydrase, this reaction quickly goes to equilibrium. The CO_2 thus formed diffuses into the cells and peritubular fluid. For every filtered HCO_3^- ion that combines with H^+, a filtered Na^+ ion is reabsorbed, and with it a HCO_3^- that resulted from the intracellular hydration of CO_2. The net result of this mechanism is the return of Na^+ and HCO_3^- to the peritubular fluid and blood; filtered HCO_3^- is conserved even though the HCO_3^- that is reabsorbed is not actually the ion that was filtered. It is to be noted that this is a mechanism for *reclaiming the filtered HCO_3^-*, not for excreting H^+. To the extent that the CO_2 formed within the tubular lumen returns to the cell to form more H^+, no net secretion of H^+ takes place.

It has been determined by micropuncture that the pH of proximal tubular fluid decreases by about 0.3 unit (Fig. 10-2), and that the P_{CO_2} is roughly the same as in peritubular plasma. Using the Henderson-Hasselbalch equation (Eq. 9-8), one can therefore estimate that the HCO_3^- concentration of tubular fluid toward the end of the proximal tubule is 8 to 10 mEq/liter. Combining this estimate with knowledge of the tubular fluid to plasma (TF/P) inulin (see Answer to Problem 8-1 at the end of the text), one can calculate that nearly 90% of the filtered HCO_3^- must be reabsorbed in the proximal tubule. Perhaps 2% is

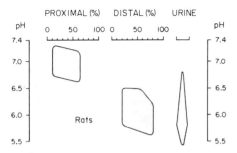

Figure 10-2
Changes in pH of tubular fluid in its course along the nephron. The enclosed areas cover the approximate range of values. Redrawn from Gottschalk, C. W., Lassiter, W. E., and Mylle, M. *Amer. J. Physiol.* 198:581, 1960; and Vieira, F. L., and Malnic, G. *Amer. J. Physiol.* 214:710, 1968.

reabsorbed in the late portion of the proximal tubule that is not accessible to micropuncture, and in the loops of Henle. About 8% of the filtered HCO_3^- is reabsorbed in the distal tubule, and only a negligible amount in the collecting duct.

Factors Influencing the Rate at Which Filtered HCO_3^- Is Reabsorbed. At least four factors can modify the rate at which filtered HCO_3^- is reabsorbed: the arterial P_{CO_2}, the concentration of K^+ in the plasma, the concentration of Cl^- in the plasma, and adrenal cortical hormones.

1. The effect of arterial P_{CO_2} is shown in Figure 10-3a. As P_{CO_2} is lowered (as by hyperventilation), HCO_3^- reabsorption is decreased, and as P_{CO_2} is raised (as by alveolar hypoventilation or by breathing high concentrations of CO_2), HCO_3^- reabsorption is increased. This effect will obviously tend to compensate the pH in a primary respiratory disturbance (see Chap. 9 and Eq. 9-8).

The mechanism that alters HCO_3^- reabsorption in response to changes in the arterial P_{CO_2} probably involves an increased intracellular supply of CO_2 substrate for the formation of H^+ and HCO_3^- (Fig. 10-1). The P_{CO_2} in peritubular blood and interstitial fluid is in equilibrium with that in the cell. Hence, as arterial P_{CO_2} is increased, that within the tubular cell also rises. Consequently, more H^+ and HCO_3^- are produced within the cell, and the entire process illustrated in Figure 10-1 is increased. Conversely, when arterial P_{CO_2} is reduced, the entire process is decreased.

2. An inverse correlation between the concentration of K^+ in plasma and the rate at which filtered HCO_3^- is reabsorbed is shown in Figure 10-3b. The mechanism for this effect may involve the movement of K^+ and H^+ across the peritubular membrane of renal cells. These events are described in greater detail in Chapter 11, where the point is made that the peritubular membrane of renal cells is roughly analogous to the serosal membrane of most body cells. As plasma K^+ is increased, either by ingesting K^+ salts or infusing them intravenously, K^+ enters cells, including those lining the renal tubules. H^+, among other cations, leaves the cells. Consequently, the H^+ concentration within the tubular cells will be reduced, and less H^+ will be secreted. Since, in the mechanism illustrated in Figure 10-1, one HCO_3^- is reabsorbed for each H^+ that is secreted, there will also be a reduction in the reabsorption of filtered HCO_3^-. The converse chain of events presumably occurs when the plasma K^+ concentration is reduced, as by curtailing K^+ intake.

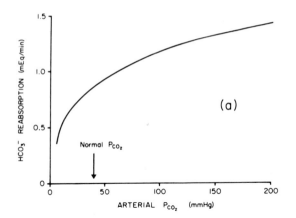

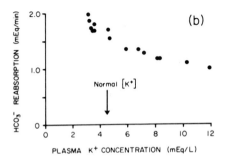

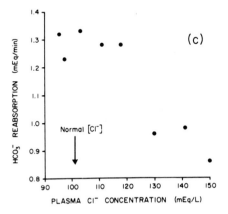

Figure 10-3

(a) Changes in the rate of HCO$_3^-$ reabsorption in dogs as the arterial P$_{CO_2}$ is either lowered through hyperventilation or raised through breathing gas mixtures containing increased concentrations of CO$_2$. Adapted from Rector, F. C., Jr., et al. *J. Clin. Invest.* 39:1706, 1960.

(b) Changes in the rate of HCO$_3^-$ reabsorption in dogs as the plasma K$^+$ concentration is varied through the intravenous infusion of K$^+$ salts. Data from Fuller, G. R., MacLeod, M. B., and Pitts, R. F. *Amer. J. Physiol.* 182:111, 1955.

(c) Influence of the plasma Cl$^-$ concentration on the rate at which filtered HCO$_3^-$ is reabsorbed. The data are from dogs in which the plasma Cl$^-$ concentration was changed through the intravenous infusion of NaCl. From Pitts, R. F., and Lotspeich, W. D. *Amer. J. Physiol.* 147:138, 1946.

This explanation may apply mainly to instances of relatively severe K^+ depletion. During mild K^+ deficit, the explanation may involve contraction of the extracellular fluid volume, for the effect on HCO_3^- reabsorption can be reversed merely by giving NaCl, without supplementing K^+.

3. There is an inverse correlation between the plasma concentration of Cl^- and the rate at which filtered HCO_3^- is reabsorbed (Fig. 10-3c). The mechanism for this effect is not fully understood. It may involve the well-known reciprocal relationship between the plasma concentrations of Cl^- and of HCO_3^-. In most situations, as the plasma Cl^- concentration falls, that of HCO_3^- rises, and vice versa; the same is true when the initial event is a decrease or increase in HCO_3^-. The explanation for this reciprocal relationship may involve the relative constancy of the total anion concentration of plasma which, given the electroneutrality of the plasma compartment, may be dictated by the primacy of a stable plasma Na^+ concentration (see Fig. 2-2).

Given this reciprocal relationship, as plasma Cl^- concentration rises, that of HCO_3^- falls. Consequently, the HCO_3^- concentration in the glomerular filtrate also falls, and since this is the acceptor for the secreted H^+ in the mechanism shown in Figure 10-1, less H^+ will be secreted. Inasmuch as in this mechanism one HCO_3^- is reabsorbed for each H^+ that is secreted, there will also be a decrease in the rate at which filtered HCO_3^- is reabsorbed.

4. An increased plasma concentration of adrenal corticosteroids, as in Cushing's syndrome, leads to increased reabsorption of filtered HCO_3^-, and the converse occurs during adrenal cortical insufficiency (Addison's disease). The explanation probably lies in the influence of adrenal cortical hormones on urinary K^+ excretion, which is discussed further in Chapter 11. A surfeit of these hormones leads to increased K^+ excretion and eventually to K^+ depletion and a low plasma K^+ concentration. At this point, the chain of events described in paragraph 2 and in Figure 10-3b would lead to increased reabsorption of filtered HCO_3^-. Thus, the influence of the adrenal corticosteroids on HCO_3^- reabsorption might ultimately involve the mechanism whereby changes in the plasma concentration of K^+ alter the rate at which filtered HCO_3^- is reabsorbed. Consistent with this explanation is the finding that the changes in HCO_3^- reabsorption that are seen in patients with Cushing's syndrome can be abolished by giving them K^+ supplements.

Replenishment of Depleted HCO_3^- Stores

It was pointed out at the beginning of Chapter 9 that in persons whose diet is fairly high in protein, there is a net daily production of nonvolatile (fixed) acids. These are mainly sulfuric acid, resulting from protein catabolism, and phosphoric acid, which is produced chiefly during the catabolism of phospholipids. These two acids are buffered by the following types of reactions:

$$2 H^+ + SO_4^= + 2 Na^+ + 2 HCO_3^- \rightleftharpoons 2 Na^+ + SO_4^= + 2 H_2O + 2 CO_2 \nearrow \qquad (10\text{-}1)$$

$$2 H^+ + HPO_4^= + 2 Na^+ + 2 HCO_3^- \rightleftharpoons 2 Na^+ + HPO_4^= + 2 H_2O + 2 CO_2 \nearrow \qquad (10\text{-}2)$$

The CO_2 is eliminated via the lungs, as indicated by the diagonal arrows, and the two neutral salts, Na_2SO_4 and Na_2HPO_4, are filtered into Bowman's space. If these neutral salts were excreted in the urine, the body would soon become depleted of $NaHCO_3$, the main extracellular buffer that is utilized in neutralizing the fixed acids. The kidneys prevent such possible depletion of $NaHCO_3$, by two means: (a) the excretion of NH_4^+, which applies mainly to the handling of filtered Na_2SO_4; and (b) the excretion of titratable acid (T.A.), which pertains primarily to the filtered Na_2HPO_4. In both operations, HCO_3^-, newly formed within renal tubular cells, is absorbed into the peritubular blood along with Na^+ that was filtered.

Excretion of Titratable Acid (T.A.)

In this process, a neutral salt such as Na_2HPO_4 is converted to the acid salt, NaH_2PO_4. Formation of such acid salts reduces the pH of the urine; the amount of strong base required to titrate the acid urine back to a pH of 7.40 (which is normally the pH of the glomerular filtrate) is *equal to the amount of titratable acid that was excreted in the urine.*

The probable mechanism for the formation of urinary T.A. is shown in Figure 10-4. As was the case for the reabsorption of filtered HCO_3^-, so too the amount of T.A. in the urine can be reduced by inhibiting the enzyme, carbonic anhydrase (e.g., as with acetazolamide). Again, therefore, the hydration of CO_2 within the renal cell is thought to be the reaction that generates the H^+ that is secreted, and the HCO_3^- that is added to the blood. Within the tubular lumen, the secreted H^+ combines with filtered Na_2HPO_4 to form NaH_2PO_4, which is excreted as T.A. in the urine. The filtered Na^+ that is liberated in this reaction is reabsorbed into the peritubular fluid and blood, along with the HCO_3^- that was newly formed within the cell. These reactions probably occur in all nephron segments.

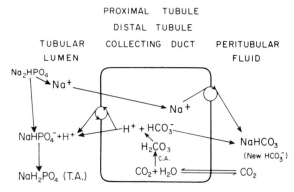

PROXIMAL   TUBULE

DISTAL   TUBULE

TUBULAR   COLLECTING   DUCT   PERITUBULAR
LUMEN   FLUID

Figure 10-4
Mechanism whereby titratable acid (T.A.) is created, and newly formed HCO_3^- is added to the blood along with a reabsorbed Na^+. CO_2 in the peritubular fluid is shown to be in equilibrium with that in the cell, to emphasize that the CO_2 substrate for the generation of H^+ and HCO_3^- is not limited to that derived from the metabolism of the renal cell. C.A. stands for carbonic anhydrase.

Factors Affecting the Rate of T.A. Excretion. Three factors influence the rate at which T.A. is excreted: the availability of urinary buffers, the pK' of these buffers, and the severity of acidosis.

1. The effect of availability of urinary buffers is illustrated in Figure 10-5a, in which an increased supply of urinary buffer is reflected on the abscissa as increased excretion of phosphate. As more buffer is made available, more T.A. is excreted.

The explanation involves a limiting concentration gradient for the transport of H^+ by renal cells. Besides HCO_3^-, inorganic phosphate is the main urinary buffer. At a pH of 7.40, at which it is filtered into Bowman's space, phosphate exists mainly as Na_2HPO_4 (see Fig. 9-5), and as the urine becomes more acid, it is converted to NaH_2PO_4, which is the main urinary T.A. The minimal urinary pH is about 4.4, probably because collecting duct cells cannot transport H^+ against a concentration gradient exceeding about 1:1,000. When this minimal pH is attained (as it was in the experiment shown in Figure 10-5a), virtually all the urinary phosphate is in the NaH_2PO_4 form, and addition of even minute amounts of H^+ would then lead to a precipitous drop in pH (see Fig. 9-5). Hence, under these conditions more H^+ can be excreted as T.A. only if more phosphate is filtered, i.e., only if the availability of more phosphate buffer enables the acceptance of more H^+ without a further drop in pH. This was accomplished by raising the plasma phosphate concentration, and is reflected in the steadily increasing phosphate excretion on the abscissa.

2. A buffer is most effective within ± 1.0 pH unit of its pK$'$ (Fig. 9-5). Hence, given the normal pH of glomerular filtrate of about 7.4, phosphate with a pK$'$ of 6.8 can initially accept much more H$^+$ per unit drop in tubular fluid pH than can another buffer with a lower pK$'$ (Fig. 9-5). Furthermore, if the pK$'$ of the other buffer is close to the minimal urinary pH of 4.4, the total amount of H$^+$ that that buffer can accept over the normal range of tubular fluid pH will be less than the amount accepted by phosphate. This fact is illustrated in Figure 10-5b. Per millimole of buffer in the urine, more H$^+$ can be excreted as T.A. when phosphate is the main urinary buffer than when creatinine, with a pK$'$ of 4.97, is the main urinary buffer.

3. The influence of the severity of acidosis is shown in Figure 10-5c. At any given rate of buffer excretion, the rate of T.A. excretion is greater in acidosis than in a state of normal H$^+$ balance. The reason for this fact is not known. It is possible that it involves a decrease in intracellular pH during acidosis, including that of renal tubular cells. The increase in intracellular H$^+$ concentration may result in an increased H$^+$ concentration difference between tubular cells and lumen, which might then lead to enhanced H$^+$ secretion.

Excretion of Ammonium — Nonionic Diffusion

If the formation of T.A. were the only mechanism for excreting H$^+$, the amount of H$^+$ that could be eliminated in the urine would be severely limited by the amount of phosphate that is filtered. As soon as the titration curve for phosphate would shift to the formation of H$_3$PO$_4$, urinary pH would fall below 4.4 (Fig. 9-5) and no more H$^+$ could be secreted by the renal tubular cells. Yet, it can be shown that much more H$^+$ than that which appears as T.A. can be excreted in the urine even though the urine pH does not fall below the minimum value of 4.4. It was therefore apparent that an additional mechanism existed for the excretion of H$^+$.

The observation that in acidosis there is a rise not only in urinary T.A. but also in urinary NH$_4^+$ raised the suspicion that NH$_3$ might be the additional acceptor for H$^+$, as by the following type of reaction:

$$H^+ + Cl^- + NH_3 \rightleftharpoons NH_4^+ + Cl^- \qquad (10\text{-}3)$$

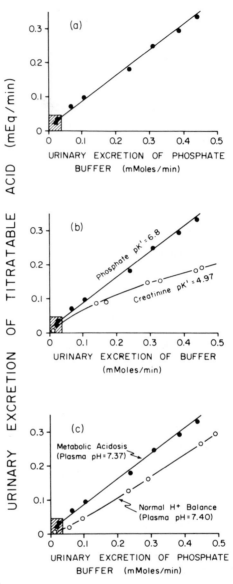

Figure 10-5
Three experiments in man, illustrating factors that influence the rate at which titratable acid (T.A.) is excreted in the urine. All experiments were done on the same person, who was either in a state of normal H^+ balance or in metabolic acidosis induced by ingesting NH_4Cl. This salt leads to acidosis through a net addition of hydrochloric acid:

$$2 NH_4Cl + CO_2 \rightleftharpoons 2 HCl + H_2O + CO (NH_2)_2 .$$

$$\text{urea}$$

Note that the H$^+$ is incorporated into a neutral salt, so that this reaction would satisfy the requirement of excreting H$^+$ without a further decrease in urine pH; in other words, neutral ammonium salts are not titratable acids.

The suspicion that the ammonia/ammonium system was involved was strengthened by the following findings: that the concentration of NH$_3$ is higher in renal venous blood than in renal arterial blood; that the delivery of NH$_3$ to the kidney from arterial blood is too low to account for the amount of NH$_4^+$ that is excreted in the urine; and that the concentration of NH$_3$ in arterial blood is unchanged in severe acidosis when urinary NH$_4^+$ excretion is greatly enhanced. The conclusion seemed inescapable that NH$_3$ must be produced within the kidney and that it is excreted as NH$_4^+$ in the urine after accepting a H$^+$.

The probable mechanism for the urinary excretion of NH$_4^+$ is illustrated in Figure 10-6. Again, it has been observed that the excretion of NH$_4^+$ is decreased if carbonic anhydrase is inhibited, as by acetazolamide. Hence, here too the hydration of CO$_2$ appears to be the reaction that contributes the secreted H$^+$.

NH$_3$ is derived from glutamine and other amino acids in the blood, which are broken down within the renal tubular cells. This un-ionized form is lipid-soluble and thus freely diffusible across virtually the entire cell membrane, which is composed largely of fat. NH$_3$ therefore diffuses passively down its concentration gradient into the tubular lumen. The pK$'$ of the NH$_3$/NH$_4^+$

(a) In this experiment, the subject was in mild metabolic acidosis (plasma pH = 7.37; plasma HCO$_3^-$ concentration = 14 mMoles/liter; urine pH = 4.5). The points enclosed in the shaded rectangle represent excretion of endogenous phosphate; all other points were obtained during the intravenous infusion of inorganic phosphate at pH 7.40.

(b) Differences in the amount of H$^+$ excreted as T.A., when phosphate is the main urinary buffer or when creatinine is the main buffer. The points for phosphate are those illustrated in (a); those for creatinine (open circles) are data obtained in the same subject (plasma pH = 7.38; plasma HCO$_3^-$ concentration = 13 mMoles/liter; urine pH = 5.1) when creatinine was infused intravenously instead of phosphate.

(c) The effect of metabolic acidosis on the rate of urinary T.A. excretion. The points for metabolic acidosis are the same as those illustrated in (a); those during normal H$^+$ balance (open circles) were obtained in the same subject. Points within the shaded area were obtained during the excretion of endogenous phosphate, and the remaining points during the infusion of phosphate at a pH of 7.40.

All three graphs slightly modified from Schiess, W. A., Ayer, J. L., Lotspeich, W. D., and Pitts, R. F. *J. Clin. Invest.* 27:57, 1948. It is of interest that the subject for the experiments illustrated here was Dr. Pitts, whose work has contributed so much to our understanding of the renal regulation of acid-base balance.

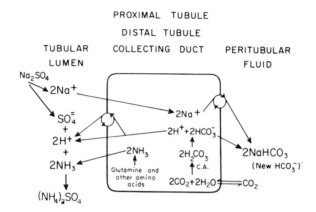

Figure 10-6
Mechanism for the renal excretion of NH_4^+. CO_2 as well as glutamine and other amino acids in the blood contribute substrates for the intracellular reactions which generate H^+, HCO_3^-, and NH_3. C.A. stands for carbonic anhydrase.

NH$_4^+$ is excreted mainly as the neutral chloride salt (see Answer to Problem 11-1 and its figure). The excretion of $(NH_4)_2SO_4$ is shown here to indicate how the filtered Na_2SO_4, which is derived from the metabolism of proteins (Eq. 9-2) and subsequent buffering (Eq. 10-1), is handled.

buffer system is about 9.2. Therefore, at the pH of tubular fluid, H^+ avidly combines with NH_3 so that the system exists almost entirely in the NH_4^+ form (see Fig. 9-5). This ionized form, unlike NH_3, is water-soluble and therefore traverses the cell membrane much less readily, since its transit is confined to the aqueous channels. Consequently, the NH_4^+ is trapped within the tubular lumen, and is then excreted in the form of neutral salts, such as NH_4Cl or $(NH_4)_2SO_4$. In the process, the HCO_3^-, which was newly formed within the tubular cell, is added to the blood along with a filtered Na^+ that is reabsorbed. As was the case with the excretion of T.A. the net result of the NH_4^+ mechanism is thus the excretion of H^+, the replenishment of the body HCO_3^- stores, and the reabsorption of filtered Na^+. These reactions probably occur in all segments of the nephron.

Nonionic Diffusion. The process by which the lipid-soluble moiety of a buffer pair (e.g., NH_3) can readily diffuse across a cell membrane, while the water-soluble member (e.g., NH_4^+) cannot, is known as nonionic diffusion or diffusion-trapping. Note that in the case of the urinary excretion of NH_4^+ this process aids the secretion of NH_3 and hence the excretion of H^+. The moment that NH_3 enters the tubular lumen, virtually all of it is converted to NH_4^+, so that a constant "sink" for the continued diffusion of NH_3 is maintained. This positive feedback, so to speak, is the more effective, the lower the urine pH; i.e., the secretion of NH_3, and hence the excretion of H^+, are most efficient in acidosis when more H^+ needs to be eliminated.

Nonionic diffusion is a common biological phenomenon that has important clinical applications in promoting the urinary excretion of weak acids and weak bases. An example of the utilization of this principle in the treatment of phenobarbital poisoning is given in Problem 10-1 and the corresponding Answer.

Control of Renal NH_3 Production and Excretion. At least three factors influence the amount of NH_3 that is produced and secreted into the tubular lumen: the pH of the urine, the degree of acidosis, and the relative rates of flow of peritubular blood and tubular fluid.

1. The influence of urine pH was discussed above and is depicted in Figure 10-7. During both normal H^+ balance and states of metabolic acidosis, there is an inverse relationship between the urine pH and the amount of total ammonia (i.e.,

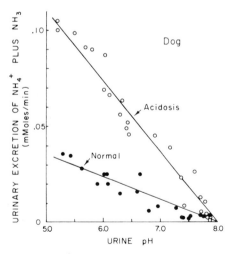

Figure 10-7
Influence of urine pH and state of acid-base balance, on the urinary excretion of total ammonia (NH_4^+ plus NH_3). All the data were obtained from one dog. At the beginning of each experiment the urine pH was about 5.2, both in normal H^+ balance and during metabolic acidosis. The urine pH was then gradually increased in each instance by infusing $NaHCO_3$ intravenously. From Pitts, R. F. *Fed. Proc.* 7:418, 1948.

NH_3 plus NH_4^+) that is excreted in the urine. The more acid the urine, the greater the proportion of total ammonia that exists in the ionized form; hence, the more acid the urine, the lower the urinary concentration of NH_3 and the greater the concentration difference promoting the passive diffusion of NH_3 from renal tubular cell into the tubular lumen. Since this NH_3 is immediately converted to NH_4^+ within the tubular lumen, it cannot diffuse back into the cell, but is instead excreted.

2. The influence of the severity of acidosis is also illustrated in Figure 10-7, which shows that, *at any given urine pH,* the rate of total ammonia excretion is higher in acidosis than during normal H^+ balance. It is important to note that this does not involve the explanation given in paragraph 1., since the difference can be detected at the same urine pH. Almost certainly the explanation involves an increased renal production of NH_3, which is an important adaptive mechanism that enables increased excretion of H^+ during acidosis. Despite a great deal of work, it is not yet known precisely how this adaptation comes about.

3. When tubular fluid has the same pH as blood, which it usually does not (Fig. 10-2), the flow rates of these two solutions determine the rates of NH_3 diffusion into them. Since peritubular blood flow is much greater than the flow of tubular fluid, blood would carry off the NH_3 more rapidly and thereby maintain a more favorable sink for the further diffusion of NH_3. Normally, however, when tubular fluid is acid, about 75% of the NH_3 produced within renal cells diffuses into the tubular lumen, and about 25% into the blood. Under the admittedly unusual conditions, when the pH of the two fluids is equal, or when the pH is higher in tubular fluid than in blood, the majority of renal NH_3 diffuses into the blood.

Relative Excretion Rates of Titratable Acid and Ammonium

Table 10-1 shows rates of H^+ excretion as NH_4^+ and as T.A., both in the normal situation and in two disease states that are characterized by disturbances of H^+ balance. It was pointed out in the beginning of Chapter 9 that in a normal person whose diet is relatively high in protein, there is a net daily production of 40 to 60 mMoles of fixed acids. In the steady (equilibrium) state, this amount of acid is excreted as H^+ combined either with NH_3 or as T.A. Since the major portion of the daily fixed acid load is H_2SO_4, which is ultimately excreted as NH_4^+ (see legend to Fig. 10-6), more H^+ is normally excreted as NH_4^+ than as T.A.

During uncontrolled diabetes mellitus, there is an overproduction of fixed acids, mainly β-OH butyric acid. This leads to

Table 10-1
Relative excretion rates of ammonium and titratable acid (T.A.) in normal man and in two disease states that are accompanied by primary metabolic acidosis. From Pitts, R. F. *Science* 102:49;81, 1945. Published with permission.

Condition	mEq of urinary H^+ per day
Normal man	
H^+ combined with NH_3	30 to 50
H^+ as T.A.	10 to 30
Diabetic acidosis	
H^+ combined with NH_3	300 to 500
H^+ as T.A.	75 to 250
Chronic renal disease	
H^+ combined with NH_3	0.5 to 15
H^+ as T.A.	2 to 20

primary metabolic acidosis which, as discussed earlier, increases the urinary excretion of both T.A. (Fig. 10-5c) and NH_4^+ (Fig. 10-7). The pK' of β-OH butyrate is slightly less than that of creatinine; hence β-OH butyrate is ordinarily a less effective urinary buffer than are phosphate and creatinine (Fig. 10-5b). During diabetic acidosis, however, the endogenous production, and hence the filtered load of β-OH butyrate, are so great that in this condition β-OH butyrate is the main urinary buffer, and T.A. appears primarily as β-OH butyric acid. Nevertheless, the data in Table 10-1 during diabetic acidosis show that the potential supply of NH_3 as a urinary buffer is considerably greater than that of buffers that form titratable acids.

During chronic renal disease, which is accompanied by a marked decrease in the amount of functioning renal tissue, there may be a reduction in both forms of fixed acid excretion, depending largely on the protein content of the patient's diet. The reduction, however, is relatively much greater for NH_3 than for T.A. This is so because the rate of T.A. excretion depends largely on the urinary excretion of buffer (Fig. 10-5a), which may remain normal until very advanced renal disease; formation of NH_4^+, however, depends on the renal cellular production of NH_3, which is greatly curtailed as the amount of functioning renal tissue is reduced.

Summary

The kidneys play a major role in the regulation of H^+ balance by maintaining the normal body store (and hence concentration) of

HCO_3^-, and by excreting the H^+ that is derived from the daily production of noncarbonic (fixed) acids. Preservation of the HCO_3^- store is accomplished through: (a) the reabsorption of virtually all the HCO_3^- that is filtered; and (b) the formation of new HCO_3^- within renal cells and addition of this HCO_3^- to the blood. Net excretion of H^+ also occurs via two mechanisms: (c) the excretion of titratable acid (T.A.), which is quantified as the amount of strong base that must be added to acid urine in order to return its pH to 7.40; and (d) the excretion of neutral NH_4^+ salts after H^+ has combined with secreted NH_3. The last process involves the principle of nonionic diffusion or diffusion-trapping.

Process (a) above is illustrated in Figure 10-1. Process (b) occurs as part of the mechanisms whereby T.A. and NH_4^+ are formed; these are depicted in Figures 10-4 and 10-6, respectively. The rate at which filtered HCO_3^- is reabsorbed is affected by: the arterial P_{CO_2}, the plasma K^+ concentration, the plasma Cl^- concentration, and adrenal cortical hormones. The rate of T.A. excretion is influenced by: the availability of urinary buffers, the pK' of these buffers, and the degree of acidosis. And the rate of urinary NH_4^+ excretion is governed by: the urine pH, the severity of acidosis, and by the relative flow rates of peritubular blood and tubular fluid, especially when the urine pH is equal to or higher than the plasma pH.

Normally, about three-fourths of the daily endogenous load of fixed acid is excreted as NH_4^+, and the remainder as T.A. The potential supply of NH_3 as a H^+ acceptor is very large, rising as much as tenfold in states such as diabetic acidosis. Since NH_3 is generated within renal cells, however, this adaptive mechanism may be greatly curtailed in chronic renal disease, when the total amount of functioning renal tissue is reduced.

Problem 10-1   *Utilization of the Principle of Nonionic Diffusion in the Treatment of Phenobarbital Poisoning.*   A 23-year-old woman is admitted to the emergency ward in coma and with a history of having ingested a large amount of phenobarbital. Her respirations are shallow, and her systemic blood pressure is somewhat low. The patient is several times incontinent of urine, which probably means that urine production is adequate despite the mild hypotension.

After instituting measures to re-establish normal respiration and to support the systemic circulation, the attending physician begins efforts to hasten the excretion of phenobarbital. Although much of the drug is metabolized in the liver, as much as 30% of the total dose may be excreted unchanged by the kidney. The compound enters the tubular system mainly through filtration, and it is then passively reabsorbed. Many physicians would choose to treat this patient by means of dialysis, either with an artificial kidney or through peritoneal dialysis. When the urine flow is adequate, however, as in this patient, forced diuresis with alkalinization is an acceptable alternate mode of therapy.

The attending physician therefore begins to infuse mannitol and $NaHCO_3$ intravenously. Mannitol is freely filtered but very poorly or not at all reabsorbed. Hence, by contributing to the osmolality of tubular fluid, mannitol inhibits the passive reabsorption of water, and initiates a diuresis. By this means, mannitol decreases the passive reabsorption of phenobarbital, analogous to the reduction of passive urea reabsorption when the urine flow is increased (see Chap. 4). The infusion of $NaHCO_3$ will alkalinize the urine and thereby diminish the passive reabsorption of the weak acid, phenobarbital, through the process of nonionic diffusion.

It is determined that the concentration of total phenobarbital (i.e., the un-ionized plus the ionized form) in this patient is 10 mg per 100 ml of plasma. About 40% of phenobarbital is bound to plasma proteins. On admission, the plasma pH is 7.3 (primary respiratory acidosis due to depression of the respiratory center) and urine pH is 5.2; after correcting the alveolar hypoventilation through assisted respiration, and infusing $NaHCO_3$, the plasma pH is 7.7 and the urine pH is 8.2. The pK' of the phenobarbital system is 7.2. Given these facts, complete the table below.

	Total Unbound Phenobarbital in Plasma (mg/100 ml)	Ratio of Unbound Phenobarbital: $\dfrac{[Ionized]}{[Un\text{-}ionized]}$	Plasma Concentration of Unbound Phenobarbital Ionized Un-ionized (mg/100 ml)
Plasma, pH 7.3			
Plasma, pH 7.7			
Urine, pH 5.2			
Urine, pH 8.2			

Selected References

General

Christensen, H. N. *Body Fluids and the Acid-Base Balance.* Saunders, Philadelphia, 1964. (A programmed text.)

Masoro, E. J., and Siegel, P. D. *Acid-Base Regulation: Its Physiology and Pathophysiology.* Saunders, Philadelphia, 1971.

Pitts, R. F. *Mechanisms for Stabilizing the Alkaline Reserves of the Body.* The Harvey Lectures, Series XLVIII, 1952–53. Academic, New York, 1954.

Pitts, R. F. *Physiology of the Kidney and Body Fluids.* Year Book, 2d ed., Chicago, 1968.

Rector, F. C., Jr. Renal Secretion of Hydrogen. In C. Rouiller and A. F. Muller (Eds.), *The Kidney,* vol. III. Academic, New York, 1971.

Rector, F. C., Jr. (Ed.). Symposium on Acid-Base Homeostasis. *Kidney Int.* 1:273, 1972.

Steinmetz, P. R. Excretion of acid by the kidney: Functional organization and cellular aspects of acidification. *New Eng. J. Med.* 278:1102, 1968.

H^+ Secretion

Gottschalk, C. W., Lassiter, W. E., and Mylle, M. Localization of urine acidification in the mammalian kidney. *Amer. J. Physiol.* 198:581, 1960.

Malnic, G., and Giebisch, G. Mechanism of renal hydrogen ion secretion. *Kidney Int.* 1:280, 1972.

Malnic, G., Mello-Aires, M., and Giebisch, G. Micropuncture study of renal tubular hydrogen ion transport during alterations of acid-base equilibrium in the rat. *Amer. J. Physiol.* 222:147, 1972.

Steinmetz, P. R. Acid-base relations in epithelium of turtle bladder: Site of active step in acidification and role of metabolic CO_2. *J. Clin. Invest.* 48:1258, 1969.

Steinmetz, P. R., Omachi, R. S., and Frazier, H. S. Independence of hydrogen ion secretion and transport of other electrolytes in turtle bladder. *J. Clin. Invest.* 46:1541, 1967.

Vieira, F. L., and Malnic, G. Hydrogen ion secretion by rat renal cortical tubules as studied by an antimony microelectrode. *Amer. J. Physiol.* 214:710, 1968.

Conservation of Filtered HCO_3^-

Fuller, G. R., MacLeod, M. B., and Pitts, R. F. Influence of administration of potassium salts on the renal tubular reabsorption of bicarbonate. *Amer. J. Physiol.* 182:111, 1955.

Giebisch, G., MacLeod, M. B., and Pitts, R. F. Effect of adrenal steroids on renal tubular reabsorption of bicarbonate. *Amer. J. Physiol.* 183:377, 1955.

Kassirer, J. P., and Schwartz, W. B. Correction of metabolic alkalosis in man without repair of K^+ deficiency: A re-evaluation of the role of potassium. *Amer. J. Med.* 40:19, 1966.

Levine, D. Z. Effect of acute hypercapnia on proximal tubular water and bicarbonate reabsorption. *Amer. J. Physiol.* 221:1164, 1971.

Malnic, G., Mello-Aires, M. Kinetic study of bicarbonate reabsorption in proximal tubule of the rat. *Amer. J. Physiol.* 220:1759, 1971.

Maren, T. H. Carbonic anhydrase: Chemistry, physiology, and inhibition. *Physiol. Rev.* 47:595, 1967.

Pitts, R. F., and Lotspeich, W. D. Bicarbonate and the renal regulation of acid base balance. *Amer. J. Physiol.* 147:138, 1946.

Rector, F. C., Jr., Carter, N. W., and Seldin, D. W. The mechanism of bicarbonate reabsorption in the proximal and distal tubules of the kidney. *J. Clin. Invest.* 44:278, 1965.

Walser, M., and Mudge, G. H. Renal Excretory Mechanisms. In C. L. Comar and F. Bronner (Eds.), *Mineral Metabolism.* Academic, New York. 1960.

Titratable Acid and Ammonia

Balagura-Baruch, S. Renal Metabolism and Transfer of Ammonia. In C. Rouiller and A. F. Muller (Eds.), *The Kidney,* vol. III. Academic, New York, 1971.

Malnic, G., Mello-Aires, M., de Mello, G. B., and Giebisch, G. Acidification of phosphate buffer in cortical tubules of rat kidney. *Pflügers Eur. J. Physiol.* 331:275, 1972.

Nash, T. P., Jr., and Benedict, S. R. The ammonia content of the blood, and its bearing on the mechanism of acid neutralization in the animal organism. *J. Biol. Chem.* 48:463, 1921.

Pitts, R. F. The renal regulation of acid base balance with special reference to the mechanism for acidifying the urine. *Science* 102:49; 81, 1945.

Pitts, R. F. Renal production and excretion of ammonia. *Amer. J. Med.* 36:720, 1964.

Pitts, R. F. The role of ammonia production and excretion in regulation of acid-base balance. *New Eng. J. Med.* 284:32, 1971.

Pitts, R. F. Control of renal production of ammonia. *Kidney Int.* 1:297, 1972.

Pitts, R. F., and Alexander, R. S. The nature of the renal tubular mechanism for acidifying the urine. *Amer. J. Physiol.* 144:239, 1945.

Nonionic Diffusion   Milne, M. D., Scribner, B. H., and Crawford, M. A. Non-ionic diffusion and the excretion of weak acids and bases. *Amer. J. Med.* 24:709, 1958.

Waddell, W. J., and Butler, T. C. The distribution and excretion of phenobarbital. *J. Clin. Invest.* 36:1217, 1957.

11 : Renal Handling of K^+ : K^+ Balance

Potassium is the most abundant intracellular cation (see Fig. 2-2), and it plays a central role in homeostasis. Normal concentration of this ion, both within cells and in the extracellular fluid, is a critical component of some very basic processes, such as the operation of enzymes, neuromuscular function including that of the myocardium, and H^+ balance. The kidney is the major organ that excretes K^+. This fact, coupled with the importance of K^+ in general cellular function, is perhaps the reason that K^+ balance so frequently comes into play in the analysis of clinical problems in nephrology: H^+ imbalance; nephrogenic defects in urinary concentration; diuretic therapy; acute renal failure; and hypertension, among others.

Net Transport of K^+ in Various Nephron Segments

Results of micropuncture studies are summarized in Figure 11-1. Normally (Fig. 11-1a), the fraction of filtered K^+ that is excreted in the urine is considerably less than 1.0, i.e., there is net reabsorption of the filtered K^+ so that only about 10 to 20% of the filtered load is excreted. It is clear from the graph, however, that net reabsorption does not occur in all nephron segments. The fraction of filtered K^+ that remains at various sites declines in the proximal tubule, from about 0.7 at 20% of proximal length — about the first accessible site of micropuncture — to about 0.3 at 70%, the last accessible site. Only about 0.08, or 8% of the filtered K^+ remains at the first 20% of the distal tubule. Therefore, net reabsorption must have taken place in the intervening segments, and most or all of this probably occurred in the nonaccessible portion of the proximal tubule and in the thick ascending limb of Henle. As fluid courses through the distal tubule, there is net secretion, for the fraction of filtered K^+ rises from a mean of about 0.08 to about 0.3. Events in the collecting duct can be roughly inferred from the difference between urine and fluid collected from the late portion of the distal tubule. The fact that the mean fraction in the urine is lower than the mean in

Most absorbed here

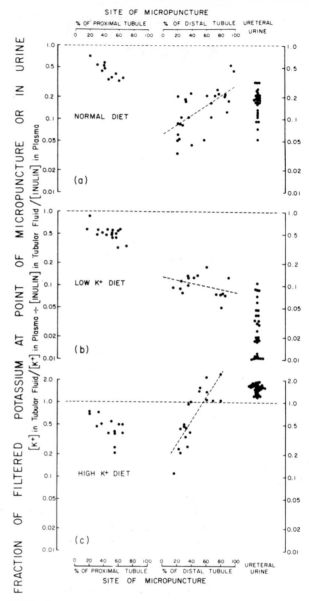

Figure 11-1

Net transport of K⁺ in various nephron segments, as revealed by micropuncture studies in rats on different diets. A negative slope of the points reflects reabsorption, a positive slope secretion. When the points for ureteral urine lie below the interrupted horizontal lines at 1.0, there has been net reabsorption of K⁺ by the entire kidney; when the urine points lie above these lines, net secretion has occurred. The site of micropuncture was determined at the end of each experiment by microdissection of the nephron. Enclosure in brackets denotes concentration. The rationale for using the concentration ratios given on the ordinate, in order to calculate the fraction of the filtered K⁺ that is found at the various sites, is explained in the Answer to Problem 8-1. Redrawn from Malnic, G., Klose, R. M., and Giebisch, G. *Amer. J. Physiol.* 206:674, 1964.

the late distal tubule reflects significant net reabsorption of K$^+$ in the collecting duct. Thus, as pointed out by G. Giebisch, urinary excretion of K$^+$ is, under a wide variety of metabolic conditions, regulated by three sequential steps: net reabsorption in the proximal tubule and loop of Henle, net secretion in the distal tubule, and a small, variable component of either net reabsorption or net secretion in the collecting duct. *SUMMARY*

As is shown in Figure 11-1b, however, net movement of K$^+$ in the distal tubule is not always in a secretory direction. When the intake of K$^+$ is low, avid conservation of K$^+$ occurs, so that only 1 to 10% of the filtered load is excreted in the urine. Under these circumstances, net movement of K$^+$ in the distal tubule is converted from net secretion on a normal diet, to net reabsorption. Note that net movement in the other nephron segments has changed very little, if at all. This suggests that modulations in net movement of K$^+$ in the distal tubule largely determine changes in the urinary excretion of K$^+$. This point is further emphasized by the results depicted in Figure 11-1c.

Net tubular secretion of K$^+$ by the entire kidney under certain conditions was simultaneously and independently demonstrated by R. W. Berliner and G. H. Mudge and their respective associates. This process is reflected in Figure 11-1c by 1.2 to 2.0 times the filtered amount of K$^+$ appearing in the urine when the animals were placed on a high K$^+$, low Na$^+$ diet. Even under these conditions, there was net reabsorption in the proximal tubule, to about the same extent as in the conditions shown in Figure 11-1a and b. Thus, even when more than the filtered load is excreted, at least 80% of the filtered K$^+$ is first reabsorbed in the proximal tubule, which process is then followed by marked net secretion in the distal tubule.

In summary, net transport of K$^+$ by the entire kidney varies with the conditions. Normally, about 10 to 20% of the filtered load is excreted, and on a low K$^+$ intake, the excreted fraction is even lower. But when the intake of K$^+$ is high, more than the filtered amount of K$^+$ may be excreted. Under all these conditions, at least 80% of the filtered load is reabsorbed in the proximal tubule. Thus, it is primarily through changes of net transport in the distal tubule — which can vary from net reabsorption to avid net secretion — that the excretion of K$^+$ is regulated.

Mechanisms of K$^+$ Transport

Reabsorption

Movement of K$^+$ across the proximal tubular epithelium is

illustrated in Figure 11-2, which is an extension of Figure 7-2. Under most conditions, the concentration of K^+ in proximal tubular fluid is slightly lower than its concentration in peritubular

PROXIMAL TUBULE

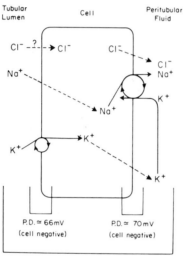

Figure 11-2
Movement of K^+ across proximal tubular cells. This diagram is an extension of Figure 7-2 and shows, in addition, proximal net reabsorption of K^+. Broken arrows signify passive transport; solid arrows, active transport via a metabolic pump.

plasma; i.e., K^+ can be moved across the epithelium against a chemical concentration gradient. Therefore, if the electrical potential difference (P.D.) across the proximal epithelium (the transepithelial P.D.) is either zero or slightly negative (see Chap. 7), there must be a component of active K^+ reabsorption. This is indicated by the "pump" in the luminal membrane. The intracellular K^+ concentration is not yet known precisely; it is probably sufficiently higher than that in peritubular fluid to permit passive movement of K^+ from cell into peritubular fluid, despite the electrical P.D. across the peritubular membrane, which tends to hold K^+ within the cell.

It was pointed out in Chapter 2 that the characteristically high intracellular K^+ concentration is maintained in part by active transport. This fact is indicated in Figure 11-2 by the attachment of K^+ to the peritubular pump for Na^+. Although there appears to be a reciprocal relationship between the movement of Na^+ and of K^+ across the membranes of most cells in the body (see Fig. 2-6), the mechanism is not a simple one-to-one exchange whereby an ion of Na⁺ is carried in one direction at the same time that an ion of K⁺ is transported in the opposite direction. For example, H⁺ as well as Na⁺ may move in a direction opposite to that of K⁺. But whatever the exchange, its location in the peritubular membrane emphasizes the point that this membrane of renal tubular cells — in contrast to the luminal membrane — may be viewed as sharing the characteristics of most serosal cell membranes in the body.

Although the distal tubule normally secretes K⁺, under certain conditions (Fig. 11-1b) it reabsorbs this ion. When this occurs, the reabsorption must be active, as indicated by the luminal pump in Figure 11-3. When the dietary intake of K⁺ is low, the concentration of K⁺ in distal tubular fluid is lower than the concentration in plasma, especially in the early distal tubule. This fact, coupled with the unquestioned electrical negativity within the distal tubular lumen relative to peritubular fluid, requires the postulation of active reabsorption. Considering the P.D. across the luminal membrane, and the chemical concentration gradient for K⁺ between lumen and cell interior, it is clear that the K⁺ pump must lie within the luminal membrane. As in the proximal tubule, so in the distal, the K⁺ concentration within the cell is sufficiently high to counteract the negative P.D. across the

DISTAL TUBULE

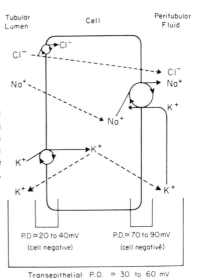

Figure 11-3
Movement of K⁺ across distal tubular cells. This figure is an extension of Figure 7-5. When there is net reabsorption of K⁺ in the distal tubule, it must be active; when net secretion occurs, it is passive.

peritubular membrane and permit passive diffusion of K$^+$ from cell into peritubular fluid.

As in most body cells, the high intracellular concentration of K$^+$ is maintained in part through active transport of K$^+$ across the serosal (peritubular) membrane.

Secretion

Net secretion of K$^+$ takes place predominantly or solely in the distal tubule (Fig. 11-1), although some secretion may continue along the collecting duct. Knowing the P.D. between tubular lumen and peritubular fluid, the K$^+$ concentration in peritubular plasma, and utilizing the Nernst equation, one can predict the K$^+$ concentration in tubular fluid that would result from passive distribution of K$^+$. Under all experimental conditions that have been tested, the K$^+$ concentration in distal tubular fluid has been lower than the theoretical prediction. This means not only that all results can be accounted for on the basis of passive secretion, but also that this passive movement is probably partially counteracted by active reabsorption from the distal tubular lumen into cell.

The magnitude of net distal tubular secretion is probably determined by three major factors: (a) the magnitude of the electrical P.D. across the tubular epithelium; (b) the concentration of K$^+$ within the distal tubular cells, which is regulated largely by the activity of the peritubular pump, transporting K$^+$ actively from the peritubular fluid into the cell (Fig. 11-3); and (c) the strength of the reabsorptive pump within the luminal membrane. That is, for any given active reabsorptive rate the more negative the electrical P.D. and the higher the intracellular K$^+$ concentration, the greater the net passive secretion of K$^+$ across the luminal cell membrane.

Factors Influencing Rate of K$^+$ Excretion

It has been known for many years that certain physiological or pathological conditions are associated with characteristic changes in the urinary excretion of K$^+$. Some of the major conditions and the associated changes have been listed in Table 11-1. Alterations in urinary K$^+$ excretion result primarily or solely from changes in the rate and/or direction of net K$^+$ transport in the distal tubule. It is therefore not surprising that the possible mechanisms listed in Table 11-1 involve mainly the factors listed in the preceding paragraph, which influence the rate of net K$^+$ transport in the distal tubule.

Intake of K$^+$. It was shown in Figure 11-1 that lowering or raising the dietary intake of K$^+$ could result in enhancement of

Table 11-1
Conditions that influence the rate of urinary K^+ excretion, and possible mechanisms through which each condition mainly exerts its influence.

Condition	Change in K^+ Excretion	Possible Mechanisms[a]
K^+ intake		
High	Increased	Increased distal tubular secretion, resulting from: Increased peritubular uptake of K^+, leading to increased intracellular K^+ concentration in distal tubular cells Greater electrical potential difference (P.D.)
Low	Decreased	Shift from distal tubular net secretion to net reabsorption, probably resulting from changes opposite to those listed above.
Na^+ intake		
High	Increased	? Decreased K^+ reabsorption in collecting duct. Increased distal tubular secretion, possibly due to ? Greater electrical P.D. ? Increased flow rate of distal tubular fluid Others
Low	Decreased	Increased K^+ reabsorption in collecting duct. Decreased distal tubular secretion, possibly resulting from changes opposite to those listed above.
H^+ balance		
Alkalosis	Increased	Increased distal tubular secretion, possibly resulting from enhanced peritubular entry of K^+, with consequent increased intracellular K^+ concentration of distal cells.
Acute acidosis	Decreased	Decreased distal tubular secretion, possibly resulting from the opposite effects.
Adrenal mineralocorticoids		
Excess	Increased	Increased distal tubular secretion, possibly resulting from enhanced peritubular uptake of K^+ and increased intracellular K^+ concentration of distal cells. ? Others
Deficiency	Decreased	Decreased distal tubular secretion, probably due to opposite changes.
State of hydration		
Deficiency of water	Increased	Increased distal tubular secretion, resulting from shift of water from intracellular to extracellular compartment, and consequent increased intracellular K^+ concentration in distal cells.

Table 11-1 (*Cont.*)

Condition	Change in K+ Excretion	Possible Mechanisms[a]
Excess of water	Decreased	Decreased distal tubular secretion, resulting from shifts in the opposite direction.
Diuretics		
Chlorothiazide	Increased	Increased distal tubular secretion, possibly due to increased flow rate of distal tubular fluid.
Furosemide	Increased	
Ethacrynic acid	Increased	
Mercurials	Decreased	Decreased distal tubular secretion, possibly resulting from decreased peritubular uptake of K+ with resultant decreased intracellular K+ concentration of distal cells.
Amiloride	Decreased	Decreased distal tubular secretion, at least partly due to decreased electrical P.D.

[a]For some conditions, the main mechanisms that have been identified are listed; for others, reasonable speculations are mentioned. The lists are not necessarily exhaustive.

net reabsorption or a shift to net secretion, respectively, by the entire kidney. These adaptations were paralleled by changes in the direction and rate of net K+ transport in the distal tubule. It is likely that the mechanism involves changes in the peritubular uptake of K+. For example, when the intake of K+ is increased, there is enhanced movement of K+ into the cell, not only at the peritubular membrane of distal cells (Fig. 11-3) but also at the serosal surface of most body cells. Other things being equal, the resulting increased intracellular K+ concentration in distal cells would then be expected to lead to enhanced passive secretion of K+ into the distal tubular lumen. The converse chain of events presumably leads not only to decreased distal tubular secretion, but even to net reabsorption of K+ in this nephron segment when the intake of K+ is curtailed.

There is another factor, at least in the chronic situation. When the diet of rats is modified for several weeks, a decreased K+ intake is associated with a decrease in the transepithelial electrical P.D. in the late distal tubule; it declines from about 60 mV in rats on a control diet, to about 30 mV (lumen negative to peritubular fluid). The opposite change occurs when rats are placed for several weeks on a diet high in K+; under these conditions the electrical P.D. at the same point in the distal tubule rises to about 85 mV (lumen negative).

Intake of Na+. In most instances there is a direct correlation between the increased urinary excretion of Na+ that follows a high intake of Na^+, and the urinary excretion of K^+. The converse also holds when the intake of Na^+, and hence the urinary excretion of Na^+, are reduced. It is important to realize, however, that there are notable exceptions, when changes in the urinary excretion of these two ions do not parallel one another. For example, administering actinomycin D to experimental animals will enhance the rate of Na^+ excretion without altering the excretion of K^+. Another example is the so-called "escape" from adrenal mineralocorticoids; when these hormones are administered for a prolonged period, Na^+ excretion returns to control values while K^+ excretion remains elevated.

The mechanisms whereby Na^+ influences the rate of K^+ excretion have not been fully identified. It is clear, though, that of all the conditions listed in Table 11-1, this is the only one in which changes in the handling of K^+ in the collecting duct, in addition to the distal tubule, make a significant contribution. Thus, during Na^+ depletion, increased K^+ reabsorption in the collecting duct is largely responsible for the low rate of urinary K^+ excretion; it is possible that opposite changes in the collecting duct partly account for the high K^+ excretion when a surfeit of Na^+ is given. In addition, changes in the rate of distal tubular K^+ secretion play a role, but the mechanisms that bring this about are not yet clear. They may include changes in the electrical P.D., and in the flow rate of fluid within the distal tubular lumen. For example, low Na^+ excretion is accompanied by a decreased P.D., which reduces the driving force for K^+ secretion. In regard to the second factor, it has been shown that under certain conditions, the flow rate of tubular fluid may be the limiting factor that determines the magnitude of distal K^+ secretion. Thus, when a solution of NaCl is given intravenously or when the dietary intake of Na^+ is high, so is the flow rate of Na^+ and hence of water in the distal lumen; this effect, in the face of a well-maintained negative transepithelial electrical P.D., enhances the rate of K^+ secretion by increasing the "sink" for K^+ diffusion into the lumen. The possible "other" mechanisms referred to in Table 11-1 include factors such as K^+ permeability and the strength of the K^+ reabsorptive pump in the luminal membrane (Fig. 11-3). The role of these additional factors remains to be assessed.

H+ Balance. Alkalosis, whether it be metabolic or respiratory in origin, is usually associated with increased urinary excretion of K^+, and *acute* acidosis of either metabolic or respiratory origin is accompanied by decreased K^+ excretion. (For reasons that have not yet been clarified, chronic states of acidosis are accompanied by increased K^+ excretion.) Figure 11-4 shows that modulations

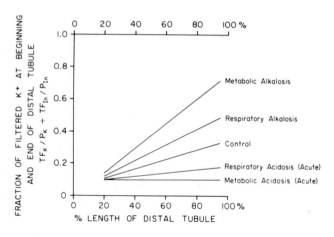

Figure 11-4
Effect of changes in H$^+$ balance on the rate of distal tubular K$^+$ secretion
in rats. The means for inducing the various states of alkalosis and acidosis
are described in the text. The rationale for calculating the fraction of
filtered K$^+$ by means of the so-called "K/In [TF/P]" is described in the
Answer to Problem 8-1. Redrawn from Giebisch, G. Renal Potassium
Excretion. In C. Rouiller and A. F. Muller (Eds.). *The Kidney,* vol.
III. Academic, New York, 1971.

in the distal tubular secretion of K$^+$ are responsible for the
changes in K$^+$ excretion. Under control conditions, the fraction
of the filtered K$^+$ rises along the course of the distal tubule (Fig.
11-1). This fraction is about 0.1 at 20% of the length — the
earliest portion accessible to micropuncture — and about 0.3
toward the very end of the distal tubule. When acute respiratory
acidosis is induced in rats by raising the concentration of CO$_2$ in
the inspired air to 15%, the rate of distal tubular K$^+$ secretion is
decreased, as reflected in the lesser slope. A similar inhibitory
effect on secretion is seen in acute metabolic acidosis induced by
an intravenous infusion of NH$_4$Cl. On the other hand, when
states of alkalosis are induced, either through hyperventilation
(respiratory) or through an intravenous infusion of NaHCO$_3$
(metabolic), the rate of distal tubular K$^+$ secretion is greatly
enhanced. The cluster of the points at 20% of distal tubular
length again emphasizes the fact that the handling of K$^+$ up to
the early distal tubule is identical under the various conditions of
H$^+$ balance.

The mechanism for the changes in distal K$^+$ secretion probably
involves reciprocal movement of H$^+$ and K$^+$ at the peritubular
membrane of distal tubular cells. It was mentioned earlier in this
chapter that the exchange of cations across the serosal mem-

branes of most body cells involves not only K^+ for Na^+, but also H^+. In states of alkalosis, the decreased H^+ concentration of extracellular fluid favors a shift of H^+ out of cells. In response to this shift, there is a net gain of K^+ by cells. To the extent that these changes occur also across the peritubular membrane of distal tubular cells, the resulting increased K^+ concentration within these cells leads to enhanced distal tubular K^+ secretion. Conversely, during acidosis, the increased H^+ concentration of extracellular fluid causes a shift of H^+ into cells and K^+ out of them, and a consequent decrease in the intracellular K^+ concentration. If distal tubular cells participate in these shifts, as they almost certainly do, the result is an inhibition of distal K^+ secretion — and hence of urinary K^+ excretion — during acidosis.

Adrenal Mineralocorticoids. Although adrenal mineralocorticoids may influence Na^+ and K^+ transport in all segments of the nephron, their major physiological effect appears to be on the distal tubule, especially on its later portions. It is mainly through adjustments in the rate of distal tubular K^+ secretion that these steroids alter the rate of urinary K^+ excretion. The effect may be mediated primarily by altering the peritubular uptake of K^+ and hence the intracellular K^+ concentration of distal tubular cells. Adrenal mineralocorticoids stimulate the "pump" in the serosal membrane of most body cells, which promotes the movement of Na^+ out of cells and of K^+ into them. Almost certainly this effect is shared by cells of the distal tubule. Hence, when there is an excess of mineralocorticoids, the intracellular K^+ concentration of distal tubular cells is probably increased, and consequently distal K^+ secretion and hence urinary K^+ excretion are also increased. The opposite effect holds when there is a deficiency of adrenal mineralocorticoids.

There may be a number of other mechanisms involved, which have not yet been identified. These might include changes in the K^+ permeability of the peritubular and/or the luminal membranes, with resultant changes in the electrical potential profile across the distal tubular epithelium.

State of Hydration. When the body sustains a loss of hyposmotic fluid — i.e., a loss of water in excess of solutes — water is withdrawn from the intracellular as well as from the extracellular compartment. Initially, water is lost from the extracellular compartment. Consequently, the solutes in that compartment become more concentrated, so that an osmotic gradient is created that favors a net shift of water from the intracellular to the extracellular compartment. This shift increases the K^+ concentration within most body cells, including those of the distal tubule. It is probably through this pathway that a loss of hyposmotic fluid — i.e., a deficiency of water — leads to an increase in distal tubular K^+ secretion and hence in the urinary excretion of K^+.

Conversely, when water is added to the body, the osmolality of extracellular fluid declines. The resulting osmotic gradient now favors a net shift of fluid into the intracellular space, so that the intracellular K^+ concentration, and hence distal K^+ secretion, are decreased.

Diuretics. The diuretics constitute a group of pharmacological agents that promote loss of fluid from the body by increasing urine flow. The chronic use of most diuretics is associated with important changes in urinary K^+ excretion.

Therapy with chlorothiazide, furosemide, or ethacrynic acid is commonly associated with increased K^+ excretion, which, if unchecked, can lead to serious K^+ depletion. Although the causes have not been fully defined, the effect may be due mainly to an increased flow rate of distal tubular fluid. This, as was discussed above under "Intake of Na^+," can lead to increased distal tubular secretion of K^+.

An increase in distal tubular flow rate is probably common to most or all diuretic agents. The fact that some diuretics decrease rather than increase urinary K^+ excretion must therefore mean that additional effects may overwhelm the influence of increased flow rate. Again, very few data that might elucidate the mechanisms of these additional effects are available. The mercurial diuretics may inhibit the peritubular uptake of K^+ and thus, by decreasing the intracellular K^+ concentration of distal cells, diminish distal K^+ secretion. It has been shown that one of the so-called K^+-sparing diuretics, amiloride, diminishes the electrical P.D. across the distal epithelium. This may be the major mechanism by which this diuretic agent completely suppresses distal K^+ secretion.

Thus, changes in K^+ excretion that accompany diuretic therapy are probably all mediated through alterations in distal tubular K^+ secretion. Both the direction and the major mechanism of the change, however, appear to vary with the particular diuretic agent.

Summary

Maintenance of a normal intracellular K^+ concentration is essential to many cellular functions. The kidney is the major organ through which K^+ is excreted; changes in the renal handling of K^+ are therefore primarily responsible for maintaining K^+ balance.

K⁺ undergoes bidirectional net transport in its course through the nephron. At least 80% of the filtered load of K⁺ is reabsorbed in the proximal tubules and loops of Henle under all circumstances. In the distal tubule, there is normally net secretion of K⁺, although this can be converted into net reabsorption in certain conditions such as K⁺ deprivation. There is usually net reabsorption in the collecting ducts. For the entire kidney, there may be either avid net reabsorption of K⁺, or net secretion. The rate of urinary K⁺ excretion can thus vary widely, and this rate is governed primarily by changes in both the direction and the magnitude of net transport in the distal tubule.

Reabsorption of K⁺ in the proximal tubule probably occurs by a combination of passive and active transport processes. In the rare instance when net K⁺ reabsorption takes place in the distal tubule, its mode of transport must be active. Net secretion of K⁺ across the luminal cell membrane in the distal segment, which is much more common, appears to be passive under all conditions. The magnitude of overall net K⁺ transport is governed by three major influences: (a) the magnitude of the electrical P.D. across the distal tubular epithelium; (b) the concentration of K⁺ within the distal tubular·cell, which is set mainly by the magnitude of active peritubular K⁺ uptake; and (c) the strength of a reabsorptive pump located within the distal luminal membrane.

Many factors — among them the dietary intake of Na⁺ and K⁺, H⁺ balance, the plasma concentration of adrenal mineralocorticoids, and diuretic therapy — can alter the rate of urinary K⁺ excretion. These alterations are brought about mainly by changing the rate of distal tubular K⁺ secretion, changes that are mediated in turn primarily by influencing one or more of the three elements listed above.

Problem 11-1   What are the urinary pH and osmolality of a healthy adult human whose diet is normal and contains protein? What are the major solutes in such urine, and what is the approximate concentration of each solute?

Selected References

General   Berliner, R. W. *Renal Mechanisms for Potassium Excretion.* The Harvey Lectures, Series LV, 1959—60. Academic, New York, 1961.

Berliner, R. W., and Kennedy, T. J., Jr. Renal tubular secretion of potassium in the normal dog. *Proc. Soc. Exp. Biol. Med.* 67:542, 1948.

Brenner, B. M., and Berliner, R. W. Transport of Potassium. In J. Orloff and R. W. Berliner (Eds.), *Handbook of Physiology.* Section 8: Renal Physiology. American Physiological Society, Washington, D.C., 1973.

Giebisch, G. Renal Potassium Excretion. In C. Rouiller and A. F. Muller (Eds.), *The Kidney*, vol. III. Academic, New York, 1971.

Kernan, R. P. *Cell K.* Butterworth, Washington, D.C., 1965.

Leaf, A., and Santos, R. F. Physiologic mechanisms in potassium deficiency. *New Eng. J. Med.* 264:335, 1961.

Mudge, G. H., Foulks, J., and Gilman, A. The renal excretion of potassium. *Proc. Soc. Exp. Biol. Med.* 67:545, 1948.

Segmental
Transport

Bennett, C. M., Brenner, B. M., and Berliner, R. W. Micropuncture study of nephron function in the rhesus monkey. *J. Clin. Invest.* 47:203, 1968.

Bennett, C. M., Clapp, J. R., and Berliner, R. W. Micropuncture study of the proximal and distal tubule in the dog. *Amer. J. Physiol.* 213:1254, 1967.

Giebisch, G., Boulpaep, E. L., and Whittembury, G. Electrolyte transport in kidney tubule cells. *Phil. Trans. Roy. Soc. London.* Series B. 262:175, 1971.

Giebisch, G., Malnic, G., Klose, R. M., and Windhager, E. E. Effect of ionic substitutions on distal potential differences in rat kidney. *Amer. J. Physiol.* 211:560, 1966.

Jamison, R. L. Micropuncture study of segments of thin loop of Henle in the rat. *Amer. J. Physiol.* 215:236, 1968.

Malnic, G., Klose, R. M., and Giebisch, G. Micropuncture study of renal potassium excretion in the rat. *Amer. J. Physiol.* 206:674, 1964.

Malnic, G., Klose, R. M., and Giebisch, G. Micropuncture study of distal tubular potassium and sodium transport in rat nephron. *Amer. J. Physiol.* 211:529, 1966.

Watson, J. F. Potassium reabsorption in the proximal tubule of the dog nephron. *J. Clin. Invest.* 45:1341, 1966.

Wiederholt, M., Sullivan, W. J., Giebisch, G., Curran, P. F., and Solomon, A. K. Potassium and sodium transport across single distal tubules of Amphiuma. *J. Gen. Physiol.* 57:495, 1971.

Wright, F. S. Increasing magnitude of electrical potential along the renal distal tubule. *Amer. J. Physiol.* 220:624, 1971.

Regulation of K^+
Excretion

Cooke, R. E., Segar, W. E., Cheek, D. B., Coville, F. E., and Darrow, D. C. The extrarenal correction of alkalosis associated with potassium deficiency. *J. Clin. Invest.* 31:798, 1952.

Cortney, M. A. Renal tubular transfer of water and electrolytes in adrenalectomized rats. *Amer. J. Physiol.* 216:589, 1969.

Gardner, L. I., MacLachlan, E. A., and Berman, H. Effect of potassium deficiency on carbon dioxide, cation, and phosphate content of muscle. *J. Gen. Physiol.* 36:153, 1952.

Gatzy, J. T. The effect of K^+-sparing diuretics on ion transport across the excised toad bladder. *J. Pharmacol. Exp. Therap.* 176:580, 1971.

Giebisch, G., and Malnic, G. The Regulation of Distal Tubular Potassium Transport. In K. Thurau and H. Jahrmärker (Eds.), *Renal Transport and Diuretics.* Springer, Berlin, 1969.

Irvine, R. O. H., Saunders, S. J., Milne, M. D., and Crawford, M. A. Gradients of potassium and hydrogen ion in potassium-deficient voluntary muscle. *Clin. Sci.* 20:1, 1961.

Malnic, G., Mello-Aires, M., and Giebisch, G. Potassium transport across renal distal tubules during acid-base disturbances. *Amer. J. Physiol.* 221:1192, 1971.

Miller, R. B., Tyson, I., and Relman, A. S. pH of isolated resting skeletal muscle and its relation to potassium content. *Amer. J. Physiol.* 204:1048, 1963.

Mudge, G. H., Ames, A., III, Foulks, J., and Gilman, A. Effect of drugs on renal secretion of potassium in the dog. *Amer. J. Physiol.* 161:151, 1950.

Mudge, G. H., Foulks, J., and Gilman, A. Renal secretion of potassium in the dog during cellular dehydration. *Amer. J. Physiol.* 161:159, 1950.

Muntwyler, E., and Griffin, G. E. Effect of potassium on electrolytes of rat plasma and muscle. *J. Biol. Chem.* 193:563, 1951.

Wright, F. S. Alterations in electrical potential and ionic conductance of renal distal tubule cells in potassium adaptation. Proceedings of the XXV International Congress of Physiological Sciences, 1971. Abstract No. 1816.

Answers to Problems

Problem 2-1   *Plasma Volume*

Equation 2-2

$$\text{Volume of compartment} = \frac{\text{Amount of substance given} - \text{Amount of substance lost}}{\text{Concentration of substance in the compartment}}$$

$$= \frac{10 \text{ mg} - 0}{0.4 \text{ mg/100 ml}}$$

$$= \frac{10 \text{ mg}}{1} \cdot \frac{100 \text{ ml}}{0.4 \text{ mg}}$$

$$= \frac{1000}{0.4}, \text{ or } 2,500 \text{ ml, or } 2.5 \text{ L}$$

Whole Blood Volume

$$\frac{\text{Plasma volume}}{55\%} = \frac{\text{Whole blood volume}}{100\%}$$

$$\frac{2,500 \text{ ml}}{55} = \frac{\text{Whole blood volume}}{100}$$

$$\text{Whole blood volume} = \frac{2,500 \cdot 100}{55} = 4,545 \text{ ml, or } 4.5 \text{ L}$$

Problem 2-2   *Total Body Water*
Again, one uses Equation 2-2

$$TBW = \frac{99.8\ g - (99.8 \cdot 0.004)}{0.2\ g/100\ ml}$$

$$= \frac{99.4\ g}{0.2\ g/100\ ml}$$

$$= \frac{99.4\ g}{1} \cdot \frac{100\ ml}{0.2\ g}$$

$$= 49{,}700\ ml,\ or\ 49.7\ L$$

Extracellular Fluid Volume

$$ECW = \frac{100\ \mu Curies - (100 \cdot 0.04)}{0.0064\ \mu Curies/ml}$$

$$= \frac{96\ \mu Curies}{0.0064\ \mu Curies/ml}$$

$$= \frac{96\ \mu Curies}{1} \cdot \frac{ml}{0.0064\ \mu Curies}$$

$$= 15{,}000\ ml,\ or\ 15\ L$$

N.B. To the extent that the distribution of sulfate between plasma and interstitial fluid is governed by the Gibbs-Donnan equilibrium, the concentration of radiosulfate will be slightly greater in the interstitium than in plasma. Since interstitial fluid constitutes about three-quarters of the extracellular compartment, the above calculation will slightly overestimate the amount of ECW.

Intracellular Volume
From Table 2-1

$$ICW = TBW - ECW$$

$$= 49.7 - 15.0$$

$$= 34.7\ L$$

Problem 3-1. Sample calculations illustrating the independence of the inulin clearance from the plasma concentration of inulin and from the rate of urine flow in a dog.

Urine Flow (ml/min)	Inulin Concentration		Inulin Clearance (ml/min)
	Plasma (mg/ml)	Urine (mg/ml)	
1.3	0.5	24	62.4
1.2	0.9	45	60.0
1.3	1.4	68	63.1
1.0	2.3	141	61.3
1.4	3.8	168	61.9
1.2	5.7	294	61.9
1.3	0.5	23	59.8
1.7	0.6	22	62.3
2.1	0.6	17	59.5
3.1	0.4	8	62.0
5.7	0.5	5	57.0
6.6	0.5	4.6	60.7

Modified from Shannon, J. A. *Amer. J. Physiol.* 112:405, 1935.

Problem 3-2. Sample calculations illustrating the identity of the inulin and creatinine clearances in a dog under physiological conditions.

Urine Flow (ml/min)	Inulin			Creatinine		
	Plasma (mg/100 ml)	Urine (mg/100 ml)	Clearance (ml/min)	Plasma (mg/100 ml)	Urine (mg/100 ml)	Clearance (ml/min)
1.0	104	5,076	48.8	13.7	673	49.1
1.1	106	4,601	47.7	14.7	630	47.1
0.9	108	6,017	50.1	16.0	890	50.1
1.0	109	5,137	47.1	16.6	792	47.7

Modified from Shannon, J. A. *Amer. J. Physiol.* 112:405, 1935.

Problem 4-1. Renal handling of inorganic phosphate in dogs.

Urine Flow (ml/min)	Phosphate Phosphorus[a] Plasma (mg/100 ml)	Urine (mg/100 ml)	Clearance (ml/min)	Creatinine Plasma (mg/100 ml)	Urine (mg/100 ml)	Clearance (ml/min)	Phosphate Phosphorus[a] Filtered (mg/min)	Excreted (mg/min)	Reabsorbed (mg/min)	Ratio: Phosphate Clearance/ Creatinine Clearance
6.8	1.25	0.07	0.4	33.9	427	85.7	1.07	0.005	1.07	0.005
6.8	1.16	0.08	0.5	32.0	392	83.3	0.97	0.005	0.97	0.006
7.0	1.02	0.08	0.5	31.3	367	82.1	0.84	0.006	0.83	0.006
9.2	2.75	0.46	1.5	31.2	283	83.4	2.29	0.04	2.25	0.018
9.7	3.70	2.95	7.7	32.5	274	81.8	3.03	0.29	2.74	0.094
8.7	4.64	9.10	17.1	33.3	321	83.9	3.89	0.79	3.10	0.203
6.7	9.34	69.0	49.5	34.5	423	82.1	7.67	4.62	3.05	0.603
7.6	11.6	83.6	54.8	34.3	375	83.1	9.64	6.35	3.29	0.659
8.2	13.0	95.7	60.4	34.5	352	83.7	10.88	7.85	3.03	0.722
9.2	23.9	171	65.8	36.9	313	78.0	18.64	15.73	2.91	0.844
10.0	27.9	184	66.0	37.7	294	78.0	21.76	18.40	3.36	0.846
10.0	31.7	208	65.6	38.7	293	75.7	24.00	20.80	3.20	0.867

[a] The values were measured as phosphate phosphorus; they have been converted from milligrams to millimoles of inorganic phosphate in Table 4-1 and Figure 4-1.

Slightly modified from Pitts, R. F., and Alexander, R. S. *Amer. J. Physiol.* 142:648, 1944. Used with permission of the American Physiological Society.

These calculations emphasize that the concept of clearance is by no means restricted to inulin or creatinine. The so-called "clearance ratio" [i.e., the ratio of the clearance of a given substance to the GFR (clearance of creatinine or inulin)] is a useful calculation in renal physiology. As explained in the answer to Problem 8-1, the clearance ratio is equal to the fraction of the filtered load of a given substance that is excreted. Thus, at a urine flow of 6.8 ml/min and a plasma phosphate phosphorus concentration of 1.25 mg/100 ml, 0.005 or 0.5% of the phosphate that was filtered was excreted; i.e., 95.5% of the filtered phosphate was reabsorbed. In contrast, at a urine flow of 10 ml/min and a plasma phosphate phosphorus concentration of 31.7 mg/100 ml, 86.7% of the filtered phosphate was excreted, and 13.3% was reabsorbed.

Problem 4-2. Handling of urea by the kidneys of adult man at varying rates of urine flow.

$\dot{V}$ (ml/min)	Urine Concentration		Plasma Concentration		GFR (ml/min)	Urea			Urea (% of filtered load)	
	Inulin (mg/ml)	Urea (mM/L)	Inulin (mg/ml)	Urea (mM/L)		Filtered (mM/min)	Excreted (mM/min)	Reabsorbed (mM/min)	Excreted	Reabsorbed
0.4	144	300	0.5	5	115	0.58	0.12	0.46	21	79
0.8	75	263	0.5	5	120	0.60	0.21	0.39	35	65
1.0	60	240	0.5	5	120	0.60	0.24	0.36	40	60
3.1	20	119	0.5	5	124	0.62	0.37	0.25	60	40
10.2	5.8	37	0.5	5	118	0.59	0.38	0.21	64	36

Problem 5-1. Determination of renal plasma flow (RPF), renal blood flow (RBF), and filtration fraction (FF), using PAH and inulin in dogs. The extraction ratio of PAH (E_{PAH}) changes during the postnatal period, during which these data were obtained.

Age (days)	Urine Flow (μl per min per g of kidney)[c]	U_{PAH} (mg/100 ml)	Pa_{PAH}[a] (mg/100 ml)	Pv_{PAH}[a] (mg/100 ml)	E_{PAH}	RPF (μl per min per g of kidney)[c]	RBF[b] (μl per min per g of kidney)[c]	C_{In} (μl per min per g of kidney)[c]	FF
2	3.8	104	2.60	2.16	0.17	898	1,633	130	0.14
21	2.7	283	1.70	1.08	0.36	1,232	2,240	270	0.22
40	5.2	664	3.00	1.23	0.59	1,951	3,547	630	0.32
60	3.2	672	1.20	0.34	0.72	2,501	4,547	790	0.32
74	2.3	3,516	3.10	0.52	0.83	3,134	5,698	1,200	0.38

[a] Pa_{PAH} and Pv_{PAH} = concentration of PAH in arterial and renal venous plasma, respectively.

[b] Assume that the hematocrit = 0.45.

[c] Values have been expressed per gram of kidney in order to correct for any changes that might be due to growth of the kidney during the postnatal period.

Abstracted from Horster, M., and Valtin, H. *J. Clin. Invest.* 50:779, 1971.

Problem 5-2
The characteristic clearance patterns are shown in Figure 5-A. The inulin clearance (U $\cdot$ $\dot{V}$/P) remains constant as the plasma concentration of inulin is increased because the numerator, U $\cdot$ $\dot{V}$, of the clearance formula increases in direct proportion to the increase in the denominator, P, the plasma inulin concentration. As the plasma concentration of inulin is raised, so is the filtered load of inulin (GFR $\cdot$ P_{In}); then, if the amount of inulin that has been filtered into the tubular system is neither subtracted from by reabsorption, nor added to by secretion, the increment in excreted inulin will equal the increment in the filtered load.

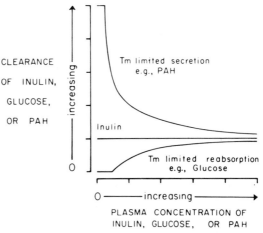

Figure 5-A
Typical clearances of substances exhibiting transport maximum (Tm), contrasted against the clearance of inulin, at increasing plasma concentrations of the substances in question. Slightly modified from Pitts, R. F. *Physiology of the Kidney and Body Fluids*, 2d ed. Year Book, Chicago, 1968.

At low plasma concentrations of glucose, the urinary excretion of glucose is virtually zero; hence, the clearance of glucose will also be zero initially. Once Tm_G has been attained, the portion of the filtered glucose that is reabsorbed becomes increasingly smaller as the plasma glucose concentration is raised (see Fig. 4-3). Stated differently, at progressively higher plasma glucose concentrations, glucose behaves more and more like inulin in that nearly all the glucose that is filtered is excreted. Consequently, at increasing plasma concentrations of glucose, the glucose clearance approaches the inulin clearance as a limiting asymptote.

The amount of PAH that is excreted is equal to the sum of that which is filtered plus that which is secreted (see Eq. 5-1). As was shown in Figure 5-1, at low plasma concentrations of PAH the secreted moiety constitutes the major portion of the total amount that is excreted. At a plasma concentration of about 65 mg per 100 ml, filtration and tubular secretion of PAH make equal contributions to the total amount excreted in the urine. Thereafter, the amount filtered becomes an increasingly large fraction of the total amount excreted, so that at very high plasma PAH concentrations, the total amount excreted will all but equal the amount filtered; that is, at very low plasma concentrations of PAH, the renal handling of PAH is unlike that of inulin, whereas at very high plasma concentrations of PAH, the handling is very similar to that of inulin, since the secreted moiety becomes negligible. Consequently, the clearance of PAH will be much higher than the clearance of inulin at low plasma concentrations of PAH, and it will approach the inulin clearance asymptotically at progressively higher plasma concentrations.

Problem 8-1. Renal handling of salt, water, and urea in varying diuretic states.

The following data were obtained on a healthy medical student, under three conditions: (a) while drinking ad libitum; (b) after 12 hours of thirsting; and (c) within 90 minutes after drinking 1 liter of tap water.

	$\dot{V}$	U_{In}	P_{In}	GFR	U/P Inulin	Proportion of Filtered Water (i.e., of GFR) Reabsorbed (%)
	(ml/min)	(mg/ml)	(mg/ml)	(ml/min)		
While drinking ad libitum	1.2	15.8	0.151	126	105	99.1
After 12 hours of thirsting	0.75	25.2	0.155	122	163	99.4
Within 90 minutes after drinking 1 liter water	15.0	1.23	0.154	120	8	87.5

Note that water diuresis is due to decreased tubular reabsorption of water, not to increased filtration. Yet, even during very marked water diuresis (15 ml/min), nearly 90% of the filtered water is reabsorbed. Also note the typical values for U/P inulin in various states of diuresis.

Problem 8-1 continued on pages 223 to 226.

Problem 8-1 *(Cont.)*

	P_{Na} (mEq/L)	Filtered Load of Na (mEq/min)	U_{Na} (mEq/L)	Urinary Na Excretion (mEq/min)	Proportion of Filtered Na Reabsorbed (%)
While drinking ad libitum	136	17.1	128	0.154	99.1
After 12 hours of thirsting	144	17.6	192	0.144	99.2
Within 90 minutes after drinking 1 liter water	134	16.1	10.2	0.153	99.1

Note that water diuresis significantly decreases the fraction of filtered water that is reabsorbed (i.e., % GFR reabsorbed), but not the fraction of filtered sodium that is reabsorbed.

Problem 8-1 *(Cont.)*

	U_{Osm} (mOsm/kg)	P_{Osm} (mOsm/kg)	C_{H_2O} (ml/min)	$T^c_{H_2O}$ (ml/min)	$U_{Urea\ N}$[a] (mg/100 ml)	$P_{Urea\ N}$[a] (mg/100 ml)	C_{Urea} (ml/min)	Proportion of Filtered Urea Reabsorbed (%)
While drinking ad libitum	663	290	−1.54	+1.54	480	12	48	62
After 12 hours of thirsting	1,000	300	−1.75	+1.75	720	15	36	71
Within 90 minutes after drinking 1 liter water	100	287	+9.77	—[b]	48	10	72	40

[a]Concentrations of urea are usually determined by measuring the amount of nitrogen in urea; hence, the expression *urea nitrogen*. The two nitrogen atoms constitute 28/60 of the urea molecule: $CO(NH_2)_2$. The clearance of urea (C_{Urea}) can be calculated without converting "Urea N" to "Urea," since the conversion factors for $U_{Urea\ N}$ and $P_{Urea\ N}$ cancel out.

[b]Note that C_{H_2O} is converted to $T^c_{H_2O}$ only when C_{H_2O} is negative.

Problem 8-1
(Cont.)

How to compute the fraction of a filtered substance that is reabsorbed. The handling of urea can serve as an example. An inulin clearance of 126 ml per minute means, of course, that 126 ml of plasma were filtered each minute. Hence, the urea contained in 126 ml of plasma was filtered each minute. The fact that the urea clearance was simultaneously 48 ml per minute means that the equivalent of 48 ml of plasma was completely cleared of urea each minute. In other words, the urea contained in 78 ml of plasma (126-48) must have been reabsorbed each minute. This amounts to 78/126 = 0.62, or 62%; and the equation for this intuitive fact is

$$\text{Fraction of filtered urea that is reabsorbed} = \frac{C_{In} - C_{Urea}}{C_{In}}$$

$$= \frac{C_{In}}{C_{In}} - \frac{C_{Urea}}{C_{In}}$$

$$= 1 - \frac{C_{Urea}}{C_{In}}$$

$$= 1 - \left(\frac{U_{Urea} \cdot \dot{V}}{P_{Urea}} \cdot \frac{P_{In}}{U_{In} \cdot \dot{V}} \right)$$

$$= 1 - \left(\frac{U_{Urea}}{P_{Urea}} \cdot \frac{P_{In}}{U_{In}} \right)$$

$$\text{Fraction of filtered urea that is reabsorbed} = 1 - \left(\frac{U_{Urea}}{P_{Urea}} \div \frac{U_{In}}{P_{In}} \right) \qquad \text{(Answers 8-1)}$$

There is another intuitive way of arriving at the same mathematical expression, through knowledge of the filtered load of urea ($C_{In} \cdot P_{Urea}$) and of the amount of urea excreted ($\dot{V} \cdot U_{Urea}$). The fraction of filtered urea that is excreted, X, can be calculated through the proportionality:

$$\frac{C_{In} \cdot P_{Urea}}{1.00} = \frac{\dot{V} \cdot U_{Urea}}{X}$$

$\therefore$ Fraction of filtered urea that is excreted $= \dfrac{\dot{V} \cdot U_{Urea}}{C_{In} \cdot P_{Urea}}$

$$= \dfrac{\dot{V} \cdot U_{Urea}}{\dfrac{U_{In} \cdot \dot{V}}{P_{In}} \cdot P_{Urea}}$$

$$= \dfrac{\dot{V} \cdot U_{Urea}}{1} \cdot \dfrac{P_{In}}{U_{In} \cdot \dot{V} \cdot P_{Urea}}$$

$$= \dfrac{U_{Urea}}{P_{Urea}} \cdot \dfrac{P_{In}}{U_{In}}$$

Fraction of filtered urea that is excreted $= \dfrac{U_{Urea}}{P_{Urea}} \div \dfrac{U_{In}}{P_{In}}$

$\therefore$ Fraction of filtered urea that is reabsorbed $= 1 - \left(\dfrac{U_{Urea}}{P_{Urea}} \div \dfrac{U_{In}}{P_{In}} \right)$ (Answers 8-1)

For the example cited above (while drinking ad libitum):

Fraction of filtered urea that is reabsorbed $= 1 - \left(\dfrac{480}{12} \div \dfrac{15.8}{0.151} \right)$

$$= 1 - (40 \div 105)$$

$$= 1 - 0.38$$

$$= 0.62$$

Answers Equation 8-1 is useful because one can compute the fraction without needing accurate urine collections; all that is required is the simultaneous determination of urea and inulin concentrations in urine and plasma. Similarly, one can determine the fraction of the filtered load of a given substance flowing at a point of micropuncture (e.g., see Fig. 11-1) without measuring the flow rate of tubular fluid; all one needs is the concentrations of inulin and of the given substance in the micropuncture sample and in the plasma.

Problem 8-2

(a) Water is probably reabsorbed in appreciable amounts from all segments of the nephron except the ascending limbs of Henle. During the formation of hyperosmotic urine, about 70% of the filtered H_2O is reabsorbed in the proximal tubules, 10 to 20% in the loops of Henle, 10 to 15% in the distal tubules, and—perhaps surprisingly—only about 1% in the collecting ducts. These figures are based on TF/P and U/P ratios for inulin, obtained through micropuncture (see Chap. 3). They illustrate at least two important points: (1) that the vast majority of filtered H_2O is reabsorbed in the renal cortex, i.e., in the proximal and distal tubules; and (2) that although the H_2O that is reabsorbed from the collecting ducts is critical to raising the urine osmolality from isosmolality to hyperosmolality, this process entails the reabsorption of relatively small amounts of H_2O.

(b) The reabsorbed H_2O must of course be immediately returned to the systemic circulation, lest the kidneys swell and burst. Almost all the reabsorbed H_2O enters the capillary beds, which are found in the cortex, the medulla, and the papilla (Fig. 1-2b). Eventually, the reabsorbed H_2O leaves the kidneys via the renal veins. An unknown but probably minimal amount of the H_2O that is reabsorbed from tubules is returned to the systemic circulation through the renal lymphatics.

Problem 9-1. The data below were obtained on each of four patients.

Normal arterial values: pH $= 7.37$ to 7.42; $[HCO_3^-] = 23$ to 25 mMoles/L; $P_{CO_2} = 38$ to 42 mm Hg.

Cause of the Disturbance	Arterial Plasma			Type of Disturbance
	pH	P_{CO_2} (mm Hg)	$[HCO_3^-]$ (mM/L)	
Prolonged vomiting	7.55	44	37	Metabolic alkalosis
Ingestion of NH_4Cl^a	7.18	28	10	Metabolic acidosis
Hysterical hyperventilation	7.57	24	21	Respiratory alkalosis
Heroin poisoning	7.07	99	28	Respiratory acidosis

^{a}The net effect of ingesting NH_4Cl is the addition of hydrochloric acid.

$$2\,NH_4Cl + CO_2 \rightarrow 2\,H^+ + 2\,Cl^- + H_2O + \underset{\text{urea}}{CO\,(NH_2)_2}$$

Problem 9-2

Respiratory acidosis. When CO_2 is retained, as during alveolar hypoventilation due to barbiturate intoxication, the P_{CO_2} rises. Since the CO_2 is buffered by nonbicarbonate buffers, it will rise at a slope approximately equal to that of the titration curve for normal blood. This is shown in Figure 9-Aa by the arrow with the dashed line going to point C. The precise slope of the straight line

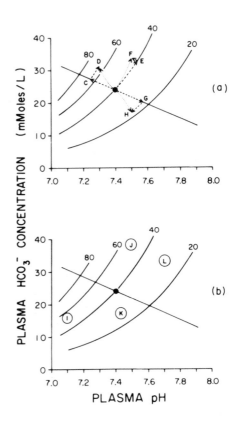

Figure 9-A
(a) Application of the pH-HCO_3^- diagram, to illustrate the dynamics of acid-base disturbances. Arrows with dashed lines indicate the theoretical major sequential steps; arrows with dotted lines indicate the probable actual paths.
  (b) Location of points representing mixed disturbances. The key for each point is given in the text.
  Slightly modified from Davenport, H. W. *The ABC of Acid-Base Chemistry,* 4th ed. University of Chicago Press, Chicago, 1958.

depends primarily on the hemoglobin concentration, and hence largely on the hematocrit. Furthermore, the actual slope—i.e., for the body as a whole—will depend on the buffer value of the composite of *all* nonbicarbonate buffers, since CO_2 quickly diffuses throughout all major fluid compartments (Fig. 9-7).

The compensatory renal response, which takes days to come to completion, is shown by the movement from point C to point D. This involves increased reabsorption of HCO_3^- (see Fig. 10-3a), and is portrayed as movement along the new P_{CO_2}

isopleth, which is determined by the deficient alveolar ventilation. The probable actual path is shown by the arrow with the dotted line.

Metabolic alkalosis. A net loss of H^+ from the body, as occasioned by the loss of gastric HCl during prolonged vomiting, is accompanied by an increase in the plasma HCO_3^- concentration (Eq. 9-10). When this occurs without a change in alveolar ventilation, movement to point E will occur along the $P_{CO_2} = 40$ mm Hg isopleth. Respiratory compensation in response to metabolic alkalosis does not invariably occur, and if it does, it is usually a slight response. This is indicated by the small arrow with the dashed line going from point E to point F; again, this runs parallel to the straight line, since it involves titration of the nonbicarbonate buffers.

Respiratory alkalosis. The primary event in this disturbance of H^+ balance is alveolar hyperventilation and a consequent decline in P_{CO_2}. Initially, this change is not accompanied by a compensatory renal response; consequently movement to point G is along the titration curve for nonbicarbonate buffers. After several days, when the renal response has led to decreased reabsorption of the filtered HCO_3^- (see Fig. 10-3a), movement to point H will have occurred. So long as the primary respiratory disturbance is not corrected, this movement will take place along the new P_{CO_2} isopleth.

Mixed disturbances. The points are shown in Figure 9-Ab. I, respiratory acidosis plus metabolic acidosis; J, respiratory acidosis plus metabolic alkalosis; K, respiratory alkalosis plus metabolic acidosis; and L, respiratory alkalosis plus metabolic alkalosis.

Problem 10-1   The Henderson-Hasselbalch equation, being an expression of the ionization or dissociation properties of acids and bases, can be utilized to solve this problem.

$$pH = pK' + \log \frac{[\text{base; i.e., } H^+ \text{ acceptor}]}{[\text{acid; i.e., } H^+ \text{ donor}]}$$

For phenobarbital,

$$pH = 7.2 + \log \frac{[\text{Ionized form}]}{[\text{Un-ionized form}]}$$

Plasma, pH 7.3

$$7.3 = 7.2 + \log \frac{[\text{Ionized form}]}{[\text{Un-ionized form}]}$$

$$0.1 = \log \frac{[\text{Ionized form}]}{[\text{Un-ionized form}]}$$

$$\therefore \frac{[\text{Ionized form}]}{[\text{Un-ionized form}]} = \frac{1.26}{1}$$

The concentration of total unbound phenobarbital is 6.0 mg/100 ml plasma; $\frac{1.26}{2.26}$ of this total exists in the ionized form, and $\frac{1.00}{2.26}$ of the total exists in the un-ionized form. Hence:

$$[\text{Ionized form}] = \frac{1.26}{2.26} \cdot 6.0 = 3.3 \text{ mg/100 ml}$$

$$[\text{Un-ionized form}] = \frac{1.00}{2.26} \cdot 6.0 = 2.7 \text{ mg/100 ml}$$

Plasma, pH 7.7

$$7.7 = 7.2 + \log \frac{[\text{Ionized form}]}{[\text{Un-ionized form}]}$$

$$0.5 = \log \frac{[\text{Ionized form}]}{[\text{Un-ionized form}]}$$

$$\therefore \frac{[\text{Ionized form}]}{[\text{Un-ionized form}]} = \frac{3.16}{1}$$

$$\therefore [\text{Ionized form}] = \frac{3.16}{4.16} \cdot 6.0 = 4.6 \text{ mg/100 ml plasma}$$

$$[\text{Un-ionized form}] = \frac{1.00}{4.16} \cdot 6.0 = 1.4 \text{ mg/100 ml plasma}$$

Urine, pH 5.2

$$5.2 = 7.2 + \log \frac{[\text{Ionized form}]}{[\text{Un-ionized form}]}$$

$$-2.0 = \log \frac{[\text{Ionized form}]}{[\text{Un-ionized form}]}$$

$$2.0 = \log \frac{[\text{Un-ionized form}]}{[\text{Ionized form}]}$$

$$\therefore \frac{[\text{Un-ionized form}]}{[\text{Ionized form}]} = \frac{100}{1}$$

i.e., when the reaction of the urine is acid, most of the phenobarbital exists in the un-ionized form which can diffuse across the membranes of tubular cells and hence can be passively reabsorbed.

Urine, pH 8.2

$$8.2 = 7.2 + \log \frac{[\text{Ionized form}]}{[\text{Un-ionized form}]}$$

$$1.0 = \log \frac{[\text{Ionized form}]}{[\text{Un-ionized form}]}$$

$$\therefore \frac{[\text{Ionized form}]}{[\text{Un-ionized form}]} = \frac{10}{1}$$

i.e., when the reaction of the urine is alkaline, most of the phenobarbital exists in the ionized form, to which renal tubular cells are relatively impermeable. Hence, alkalinization of the urine can significantly diminish the reabsorption and thus enhance the renal excretion of a weak acid, such as phenobarbital.

Note that alkalinization may have a further advantage. Giving NaHCO$_3$ alkalinizes not only the urine but also the plasma. This change reduces the concentration of the un-ionized form in plasma. Since this is the form that passes most readily across cell membranes, including those of the brain, alkalinization probably reduces the concentration of phenobarbital in cerebral cells, and thereby hastens the recovery from coma.

The beneficial effects of increased urine flow and alkalinization during experimental phenobarbital intoxication were presented in the following paper: Waddell, W. J., and Butler, T. C. The distribution and excretion of phenobarbital. *J. Clin. Invest.* 36:1217, 1957.

	Total Unbound Phenobarbital in Plasma (mg/100 ml)	Ratio of Unbound Phenobarbital: $\dfrac{[\text{Ionized}]}{[\text{Un-ionized}]}$	Plasma Concentration of Unbound Phenobarbital	
			Ionized (mg/100 ml)	Un-ionized (mg/100 ml)
Plasma, pH 7.3	6.0	$\dfrac{1.26}{1}$	3.3	2.7
Plasma, pH 7.7	6.0	$\dfrac{3.16}{1}$	4.6	1.4
Urine, pH 5.2	—	$\dfrac{1}{100}$	—	—
Urine, pH 8.2	—	$\dfrac{10}{1}$	—	—

Problem 11-1   The variation in the normal values is so great that it is almost meaningless to give average figures; hence the ranges are given in Table 11-A. When an individual is in balance (the steady state),

Table 11-A
Composition of the urine of a normal adult human whose diet includes protein.

pH	5.0 to 7.0
Osmolality	500 to 800 mOsm/kg H_2O
Na^+	50 to 130 mEq/L
K^+	20 to 70 mEq/L
NH_4^+	30 to 50 mEq/L
Ca^{++}	5 to 12 mEq/L
Mg^{++}	2 to 18 mEq/L
Cl^-	50 to 130 mEq/L
$H_2PO_4^-$	20 to 40 mEq/L[a]
$SO_4^=$	30 to 45 mEq/L
Organic acids	10 to 25 mM/L[a]
Urea	200 to 400 mM/L
Creatinine	6 to 20 mM/L

[a]At an acid urinary pH of 6.0 or lower, nearly all of the urinary inorganic phosphate exists in the monovalent form (Fig. 9-5). Urinary organic acids (e.g., lactic, uric, citric, pyruvic acids) have different valences; the molar concentration listed assumes an average valence of minus two.

the daily output of various substances (both renal and extrarenal) equals the daily production of those substances (both exogenous and endogenous). For a solute such as Na^+, which normally is excreted almost exclusively by the kidneys, the urinary *concentration* therefore depends not only on the intake of Na^+ but also on the intake of water. It is because the intakes of both solute and solvent can vary greatly from day to day that normal urinary concentrations have such wide ranges.

Note that a healthy individual whose diet contains proteins (i.e., a diet that yields fixed acids), excretes urine with an acid pH. Note also that he normally excretes urine which is hyperosmotic to plasma.

The major solutes which contribute to the osmolality of normal urine are depicted in Figure 11-A. Quantitatively, the

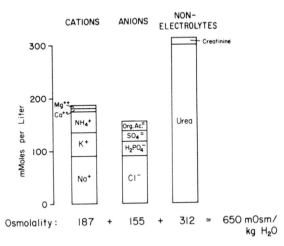

Osmolality :   187   +   155   +   312   ≈   650 mOsm/ kg H₂O

Figure 11-A
Solute concentrations of normal urine. Note that the concentrations have been expressed as mMoles per liter. Since urine contains more divalent anions than cations, the column for the anions is lower than that for cations. If the concentrations were given as milliequivalents per liter, the two columns would of course be of equal height.

most important electrolytes are Na^+, K^+, NH_4^+, and Cl^- (HCO_3^- is normally "absent"). Urea is the most abundant nonelectrolyte, and it ordinarily constitutes 40 to 50% of the total osmolality. (The reason for the inequality of the columns for cations and anions is given in the legend to Figure 11-A.)

Index